Contributions to Gynecology and Obstetrics

Vol. 7

Series Editor
P.J. Keller, Zürich

S. Karger · Basel · München · Paris · London · New York · Sydney

Surgical Geriatric Gynecology

A Contribution to Geriatric Gynecology with
Particular Consideration of
Postoperative Mortality

V. Jalůvka

Department of Gynecology and Obstetrics, Klinikum Steglitz,
Free University of Berlin, Berlin

66 tables, 1980

S. Karger · Basel · München · Paris · London · New York · Sydney

Contributions to Gynecology and Obstetrics

Vol. 1: E. Reinold (Wien): Ultrasonics in Early Pregnancy. Diagnostic Scanning and Fetal Motor Activity
VI + 148 p., 30 fig., 21 tab., 1976. ISBN 3–8055–2332–7
Vol. 2: Biochemical Methods for Monitoring Risk Pregnancies. P.J. Keller, Zürich (ed.)
X + 206 p., 86 fig., 36 tab., 1976. ISBN 3–8055–2386–6
Vol. 3: The Risk at Delivery. G.P. Mandruzzato, Trieste (ed.)
VI + 162 p., 70 fig., 75 tab., 1977. ISBN 3–8055–2421–8
Vol. 4: Female Infertility. P.J. Keller, Zürich (ed.)
VI + 146 p., 52 fig., 11 tab., 1978. ISBN 3–8055–2791–8
Vol. 5: Fetal Endocrinology. T. Zondek and L.H. Zondek, London (eds.)
X + 158 p., 39 fig., 7 tab., 1979. ISBN 3–8055–2926–0
Vol. 6: Real-Time Ultrasound in Perinatal Medicine. R. Chef, Charleroi (ed.)
VIII + 160 p., 112 fig., 18 tab., 1979. ISBN 3–8055–2976–7

National Library of Medicine, Cataloging in Publication
Jalůvka, V.
Surgical geriatric gynecology : a contribution to geriatric gynecology with particular consideration of postoperative mortality / V. Jalůvka. – –
Basel ; New York : Karger, 1980
(Contributions to gynecology and obstetrics ; v. 7)
1. Genital Diseases, Female – surgery   2. Genital Diseases, Female – in old age
3. Postoperative Complications – in old age
I. Title   II. Series
W1 C0778RG v. 7   WP 660 J26s
ISBN 3–8055–3070–6

© Copyright 1980 by S. Karger AG, 4011 Basel (Switzerland), Arnold-Böcklin-Strasse 25
Printed in Switzerland by Thür AG Offsetdruck, Pratteln
ISBN 3–8055–3070–6

Contents

Acknowledgements

Special thanks are due to Professor *Georg Hörmann,* M.D., for his constant support and encouragement. He gave me the benefit of his great clinical knowledge, thus enabling me to examine the present operation material critically with respect to the indications. I thank Dipl.-Phys. *Jürgen Pachaly* for his help in familiarizing me with electronic data processing. The present study was only possible with the help of the head physicians of 17 West Berlin gynecological departments. I am most grateful to them for agreeing that the surgical results of their departments be included in this study. I wish to thank Dipl.-Biol. *D.J. Williams,* B.Sc., for his excellent cooperation in preparing the translation into English. I also wish to express my sincere appreciation and gratitude to Professor *Paul J. Keller,* M.D., for his valuable suggestions in the final shaping of the manuscript.

Introduction

Extensive pre- and postoperative care and modern aneşthetic procedures have also resulted in a widening of the range of indication for gynecologic operations for elderly patients today. This has been underscored by numerous studies dealing with surgical geriatric gynecology, most of them published in recent years. This tendency will undoubtedly continue in future years. For this reason, we consider it valuable to carry out a systematization of existing data and to compare them with our own material.

Our survey commences with a general chapter presenting individual problems of geriatric gynecology and pointing out possibilities for future clinical research. Furthermore, references about surgical geriatric gynecology are compared. The special chapter contains an analysis of material obtained from 17 West Berlin gynecological departments with special consideration of postoperative mortality. Our own previous reports on surgical geriatric gynecology constitute an integral part of this study, but are only mentioned in appropriately placed marginal notes.

General Chapter

Time Delimitation of Geriatric Gynecology

There are hardly any differences of opinion persisting today on the concepts 'menopause', 'premenopause', 'postmenopause' and 'climacteric'. The usefulness of the division into early and late postmenopause is also generally recognized. Because of the increasing life expectancy of women, postmenopause is a part of their life which is increasingly extending in length. We can thus also speak of an increasing significance of geriatric problems in our discipline. It can be seen from table 1 that a uniform interpretation of the subdivision in time of the postmenopause and period of the senium is not yet available. For example, some authors already consider that old age has begun in the late postmenopause, whereas others consider that it only follows after the late postmenopause.

According to *Stieglitz* (110) gerontology and geriatrics may already begin with the 40th year of life. He distinguishes: (1) 'the period of later maturity', 40–60 years; (2) 'the period of senescence', 60–75 years, and (3) 'the period of senility', after the 75th year of life.

Another age classification of gerontology has been suggested, e.g. in 1962, in Leningrad (118): (1) elderly people, 60–74 years; (2) old people, 75–89 years, and (3) very old people, 90 years old and older.

For us, the third group has only theoretical significance for the time being. The first two groups are practically identical with the second and third group of *Stieglitz*. We have difficulty in transferring his suggestion for the commencement of geriatrics fully to our specialty and to speak of 'geriatric gynecology' already from the 40th year of life. However, based on the concept of *Stieglitz,* one could use the term 'postmenopausal gynecology'.

The senium is uniformly taken to mean old age. However, there is still no clarity as to whether all old female patients or only especially old patients are to be assigned to the senium.

The classification of the phases of life has always rightly been based on assessment of the existing hormonal conditions in the female organism. In contrast to previous views, the late postmenopause could be taken to mean the beginning of the hypohormonal phase and the senium to mean the advanced stage of the hypohormonal phase in especially old women.

Table 1. Definition and delimitation in time of the postmenopause and senium

Author(s)	Definition
Bickenbach (17)	senium: from 60 years onwards
Hauser (50)	postmenopause: hypergonadotropic phase; senium is a general hypohormonal stage characterized by processes of aging and atrophy in all endocrine glands
Hausschild (51)	from the 60th year of life, the period of the senium follows the postmenopause
Kaiser and Daume (58)	climacteric is the entire phase of transition from sexual maturity to old age; both parts of the climacteric before and after menopause last for about 6 years; the senium following the climacteric in about the second half of the 6th decade can also be designated late postmenopause
Kepp and Staemmler (1)	for clinical reasons, the first 2 years after menopause are designated 'early postmenopause' and the following years as 'late postmenopause', which passes into the senium
Kern (2)	senium begins with decline of physical efficiency and appearance of real aging processes in the 65th to 70th year of life
Knörr et al. (3)	after menopause begins postmenopause, which is followed by senium at about 65 years of age
Kraatz (61)	one may regard old age as starting only at 80 years, but it would be better to refer to it from the 70th year of life onwards in relation to the diseases, their treatment and declining powers of resistance
Kyank and Sommer (4)	senium is designated as late postmenopause and begins at about the age of 60
Lax (5)	'climacteric and incipient menopause'; 'the late menopause and the senium'
Pschyrembel (6)	late postmenopause = senium
Schrage (8)	senium: from the 65th year of life
Staemmler (9)	for clinical reasons, one can distinguish an early postmenopause comprising the first 2 years after the end of the cyclic function from a late postmenopause; postmenopause then later passes into the senium
Stancampiano (107)	senium: from 60 years onwards
Wittlinger and Dallenbach-Hellweg (122)	subdivide the period after menopause into early (1–5 years) postmenopause, late (6–15 years) postmenopause and senium

Geriatric gynecological problems begin at the age of 65. However, even in gynecology, it is becoming more and more difficult to refer to the senium already from the 65th or even from the 60th year of life and to designate all female patients as aged women from this age onwards. The first phase of geriatric gynecology might thus approximately correspond to the late postmenopause, and the senium begin only after the 70th year of life or even later based on the view of *Kraatz* (61).

We feel this view is confirmed among other evidence also by several surgical and anesthesiological studies on the clinical evaluation of the patient material in female patients who were at least 80 years old, despite our having found this age limit in only one paper so far in the geriatric gynecological literature (305). *Davis* (29) and *Russel* (96) also underscore the value of an age breakdown among geriatric gynecological patients, when they speak of the 'gynecology of senescence and senility'.

Terminology

We have been unable to find in the literature a consistent view on the terms gerontology and geriatrics. *Maurizio* (68) was the first and perhaps the only writer so far to use the two terms with a different meaning in the title of his study 'Attuali vedute di gerontologia e geriatria ginecologica', in which he described the full problem comprehensively.

The Czechoslovak Gynecological Society organized the congress 'Gynecological Gerontology' in Prague in 1964. This term was also used by *Mayer* (70) and *Tropea* (114). In our view, it would be better to refer to 'Gerontological Gynecology'. This term is used for example by *Quaini* (88) and *Cetroni* (24), although they are analyzing gynecological diseases. This contradiction is still more evident in the title of another communication by *Cetroni* (25) 'Patologia ginecologica gerontologica'.

Rogers (94) analyzed 'Gynecological aspects of geriatrics'. *Bickenbach* (17) considered 'Geriatrics from the viewpoint of the gynecologist'. *Bradford* (21) refers in his paper 'The gynecologist's role in the expanding field of geriatrics' to an increasing responsibility of the gynecologist for elderly women. We believe that one should lay the emphasis on the increase of geriatric problems in gynecology. In none of the three studies is it adequately shown that precisely gynecological pathology should always be dealt with from the viewpoint of our speciality, as formulated for example by *Kraatz* (61) in his communication 'Geriatric problems in gynecology'. For the reasons given, the designation 'geriatric gynecology' is to be preferred (14, 26, 41, 66, 71, 75, 78, 84, 103, 109, 117).

Some authors (140, 151, 220, 228, 246, 262, 268, 301) have used the term 'gerontology' in their papers on gynecological operations in elderly women. As is well known, gerontology is considered with the physiological processes of aging, which are only rarely an indication for surgery in our specialty. One should thus use the term 'geriatrics' and refer either to 'geriatric surgical gynecology' or 'surgical geriatric gynecology' or 'geriatric gynecological surgery'. In our view, the two latter designations place the emphasis best, which is why we have used them.

General Geriatric Gynecological Papers

The paper 'Gynecologic and other complications related to an aging female population' by *Kosmak* (59) has very often been quoted as the first geriatrically orientated communication in our discipline. However, *Lorenzola* (65) was probably the first to write on gynecological diseases in elderly women. Since then, many further communications (10–125) have been published in which typical clinical pictures of geriatric gynecology have been listed and described.

Table 2. Gynecology of elderly and very old women

Gerontological gynecology	Geriatric gynecology
Morphology	*General part*
Anatomy	Symptoms
Cytology	Diagnostics
Histology	Preventive gynecological examinations
	Sociological problems
Physiology	
Endocrinology	*Special part*
Physiological functions (sex life, etc.)	Nature of disease
	Genital displacements
Sociological problems	Dystrophies and precancerous conditions
	Benign tumors
	Malignant tumors
	Metrorrhagias not due to tumors
	Inflammations
	Injuries
	Pathology of sex life
	Other diseases
	Nature of treatment
	Conservative treatment
	Surgical treatment

The most detailed compilation on the geriatric problems of our specialty was published by *Cetroni* (23) in 1952. *Davis* (29), *Durst* (32), *Hauser* (50), *Hausschild* (51), *Lock* (64) and *Russel* (96) have written a chapter on gynecology in geriatric monographs. An excellent review on 'Geriatric gynecology' by *Navratil and Reiffenstuhl* (75) is especially to be mentioned here. In the gynecological literature, we found only a monograph by *Stoll et al.* (112). In 1973, *Wittlinger* (121) qualified to lecture at a university with the paper 'Geriatrics in gynecology'. A podium discussion on 'Geriatric gynecology' was led by *Page* (78). Several papers dealing with gynecological problems in 65-year-old and older women have been published together in *Clinical Obstetrics and Gynecology* (48).

Special Geriatric Gynecological Papers

Several hundred communications appear each year in which gynecological diseases in women who are at least 65 years old are treated in some way. In order to facilitate systematization of previous literature, we present in table 2 a draft of the conception 'gynecology of the elderly and very old woman'. It is advantageous to separate the physiological process of aging from diseases in the region of the female sex organs. This would be taken into account with the terms 'gerontological gynecology' and 'geriatric gynecology'.

In contrast to papers on 'surgical geriatric gynecology', we are not able to mention all known publications because of space problems. Nevertheless, we hope to point out sufficiently with this paper the manifold gynecological problems in elderly and very old women.

Gerontological Gynecology

In the field of 'gerontological gynecology', a meticulous survey of publications in the various anatomical, gynecological and gerontological journals appears desirable in the first instance. Comprehensive compilations of anatomical, histological, electron microscopic and histochemical knowledge of alterations in the individual female sex organs due to age are still lacking. Such fundamental research would certainly be a worthwhile task. Numerous papers have been published on the cytological alterations of vaginal smears in the postmenopause and the senium.

Even hormonal conditions in the postmenopause and in the senium have already been the subject of many communications. An exhaustive description of the dynamic hormonal changes would certainly be a worthwhile task for endocrinological gynecology. We do not only mean the deepening of knowledge of physiological alterations, but also that of numerous pathoendocrinological alterations.

Not very much attention has been devoted so far to the sex life of elderly women. With the increase life expectancy and the diminution of prejudices, its significance has become more current. Without doubt representative statements are desirable here. We should take into account not only the alterations in the female genitals due to age, but also the sexual problems resulting from their pathological state.

Symptoms in Geriatric Gynecological Patients

The most frequent symptom which occasions inpatient admission is genital bleeding even in elderly and very old women. Its causes in the postmenopause and in the senium are already analyzed in various communications. We shall be dealing later with the treatment of genital displacements in elderly women. The urinary incontinence frequently associated with them constitutes not only a medical, but also a social nursing and sociological problem, especially in very old women. According to the above-mentioned problems pruritus vulvae is one of the most frequent symptoms in geriatric gynecological pathology.

Geriatric Gynecology

We open to discussion their classification according to the kind of disease. We have not undertaken a classification according to single organs. However, in this connection *Kosmak* (60) is quoted, who already in 1946 had assigned diseases of the breast to the pathology of external sex organs.

Dystrophic changes of the external genitals were always a regular component of geriatric gynecology. With increasing life expectancy, they will increase still further in importance, especially with regard to vulvar carcinoma.

Not only can a continuous rise in the number of patients with gynecological tumors requiring treatment be observed, but also their ever greater proportion in the total geriatric gynecological patient material. The treatment of benign and malignant tumors has thus developed into the central clinical problem of geriatric gynecology. With their characteristic clinical symptoms, both the benign and malignant hormonally active ovarian tumors in particular constitute a typical chapter in geriatric gynecology (323–399).

Colpitis is in the forefront of inflammatory diseases in elderly patients. Further are described a postmenopausal tuboovarian abscess, yeast mycoses in the postmenopause and the senium, and postmenopausal tuberculous genital disease. Interesting clinical pictures result in aged women in vaginal occlusion, hematometra, hydrometra, pyometra and postmenopausal endometriosis. Several authors have discussed a possible estrogen-like action of digitalis.

The diversity of clinical problems in geriatric gynecology is underscored by quoting titles from a few recent papers: pelvic relaxation in elderly women, postmenopausal palpable ovary syndrome, gymnastics for elderly women, mental problems of elderly gynecological patients, sex chromatin in elderly women after the menopause, inversion of the uterus, uterine rupture in the senium, tubal torsion in women in the postmenopause, treatment of urethral prolapse of aged women with follicular hormones, bowel hygiene in gynecological geriatric patients, chorioepithelioma in elderly women, hydatid mole in elderly women, positive pregnancy test in an 82-year-old woman, hysteroscopic examination in aged women, variations in β-glucuronidase activity in the menopause and in the senium, widening colporrhaphy in climacteric vaginal stenoses, and local stilbene preparation before descensus operation in elderly women.

Proportion of Geriatric Cases among the Total Patients

Bickenbach (17) begins his communication with the observation that the proportion of geriatric cases is not great in gynecology. Among new admissions, women over 60 years constituted only 5.8% in one year after excluding all special consultations. His realization that a relatively high percentage (twice as high as in patients of all age groups) of the women over 60 who visited the outpatient department require inpatient treatment is important: in 28.8% of the patients, surgical treatment was necessary, diagnostic intervention had to be carried out in 9.4% and 3% had to be admitted to the septic department because of infectious diseases. According to *Quaini* (88), 3.9% of the women admitted to the hospital were over 60 years old. *Glik and Soferman* (43) analyzed gynecological diseases in 235 women who were at least 60 years old: these made up 1.4% of all admissions to the Municipal Government Hospital in Tel Aviv in the years 1958–1966.

Wittlinger (120) analyses the material of the Mannheim University Department of Gynecology and Obstetrics from the years 1966–1969. The 580 patients who were at least 60 years old constitute 12.6% of the inpatient material. *Wittlinger* also points out the positive correlation between the increase of women with a gynecological malignancy and increasing age. *Škoda et al.* (105) registered 1,430 inpatient admissions of women over 60 years old from 1954–1963. This corresponded to roughly 7% of all admissions. 997 patients (70%) were 60–70 years old and 433 (30%) were older. The following incidence of individual diseases were found: 390 benign tumors (also cervical or corpus polyps and benign portio lesions), 360 genital displacements, 321 malignant tumors, 192 postmenopausal hemorrhages, 92 leukoplakias and kraurosis vulvae, 26 inflammations and 49 other diseases. The disease frequency in the two age groups was fairly constant. There was a certain shift only in the genital displacements and malignant tumors. These occurred very frequently in women over 60 years. Descensus as well as prolapsus uteri et vaginae largely affected the women of the first age group.

In the Department of Gynecology and Obstetrics in Lund, 25,408 women were treated as inpatients from 1927 to 1946. 892 patients (3.5%) were over 65 years (10). *Fernandez-Ruiz and Villa* (37) reported on 404 women at least 60 years old in the Palencia Department of Gynecology and Obstetrics who constituted 3.1% of the patient material there. *Grönroos et al.* (47) treated 458 patients who were 60 years old and older from 1950 to 1963; these made up 2.8% of the total patient material. *Hart* (49) analyzed the results of treatment in 123 70-year-old gynecological patients, as did *Sica and de Jorio* (104) in 164 60-year-old patients. In *Borkowski* (20), the 198 60-year-old and older patients made up 4.6% of the hospitalized patients.

In our opinion, analysis of the occupation of beds in gynecological wards gives a better overview of the extent of the geriatric patient material than the proportion among all inpatient admissions. With weekly analysis in our hospital from 1.1.1973 until 30.6.1973, 1,410 gynecological beds were occupied, and of these 462 were occupied by women of over 60 years (32.8%). That this figure is markedly different from the percentages of admission reported by other authors (see above) is to be explained by the very much longer hospital stays of the elderly and aged patients.

As regards the significance of 'geriatric gynecology', it is not the few percentage figures so far available which are decisive, but the general demographic situation. Without having to quote the numerous WHO and national statistics, it is clear that one must expect a further rise in the average age.

Preventive Examinations in Aged Women and Gynecological Care of Chronic Patients

Special gynecological examinations should also be demanded in hospitals for the chronically sick. *Quinlivan* (90) reports on his gynecological experience with 600 women over 60 years old which were hospitalized in the John J. Kane Hospital for the chronically sick in Pittsburgh. *Folsome et al.* (38) reports on 611 women of the same age examined gynecologically in the Bird S. Color Hospital, Welfare Island. *Mauzey and Kaknes* (232) have carried out 151 gynecological interventions in 'elderly' psychiatric patients (on 104 women between 50 and 59 years and on 47 women over 60 years old).

The proportion of very old women who take part in cancer prevention examinations is known still to be very small. This is explained both by the understandably low readiness to undergo examinations on the part of women and the not yet very pronounced interest of the gynecologists for the diseases of very old patients. By this we do not mean only the preventive examination of hospitalized and chronically bedridden patients, but on the contrary also of wider sections of the elderly female population. We have had quite positive and encouraging experience with popular lectures in old people's homes and social centers for senior citizens. A greater readiness to undergo gynecological cancer preventive examinations was afterwards discernible (56).

Extension of these examinations should be one of our most important tasks. *Farley and Wolff* (35) examined 209 women over 65 years old in 2 years in the Cancer Prevention Center of Chicago. 35% of these spontaneously reported gynecological symptoms. After specific questioning, the proportion of the women with pathological findings increased to 76%. *Schneck* (101) reported on examinations of 636 patients over 60 years old. In 26% of the cases genital displacements, and in 4.9% carcinomas of genital organs were diagnosed. The increasing importance of gerontological and geriatric problems also for ambulant gynecological care has rightly been pointed out. A similar statistical analysis of prophylactic examinations in elderly country women was undertaken by *Müller et al.* (73). Among others, *Alechnovich* (11), *Bickenbach* (17) and *Zerzavy* (125) have pointed out the importance of gynecological cancer prevention in elderly women.

In our view, one should allot one consulting hour each week especially for geriatric patients separately from the cancer prevention consultations or if possible arrange an additional consultation time. *Turkel et al.* (115) can look back on 10 years of experience in this area. Compared to the data from *Folsome et al.* (38) from the same geriatric gynecological consulting hour, they were able to carry out not only the routine examination, but also a continuous treatment.

Literature on Surgical Geriatric Gynecology

Age

The first paper on the problems of surgical geriatric gynecology has probably been written by *Reichelt* (264). In his communication 'Gynäkologische Operationen bei alten Leuten', however, he neither specifies an age limit nor does he analyze his own material. In emphasizing the advanced age of gynecological patients who have been operated on, for example *Siliquini* (278) as well as *Weed and Mighell* (312) begin the analysis from the 50th year of life and *Caresano* (152) from the 55th year. An unusual age limit of 57 years was chosen by *Nobile et al.* (246).

Table 3. Studies on 60-year-old and older female patients

Author(s)	Cases	Proportion of all operations, %
Vácha (306)	5,615	12.5
Pernecker (255)	1,550	–
Berle et al. (141)	1,514	–
Štefánik (289)	767	6.6
Bailo et al. (135b)	708	8.0
Rigó and Zubek (267)	704	–
Gierdal and Butters (176)	686	8.4
Berger et al. (140)	681	8.5
Horn et al. (184)	670	–
Ardelt et al. (131)	660	–
Randow and Riess (263)	633	10.1
Rendina and Bellomo (265)	593	–
Mussey (242)	585	–
Suonoja et al. (293)	573	–
Trnka (303)	564	9.2
Belopavlovič et al. (137)	545	–
Rieppi et al. (266)	532	11.4
Wittig (316)	528	10.2
Rusch (271)	496	–
Siliquini and Petterino (279)	479	–
Szendi and Lakatos (296)	418	–
Skiftis et al. (281)	398	12.8
von Mikulicz-Radecki (237)	392	12.2
Kolářová and Staníček (206)	375	15.5
Pócsy and Nemecskay (259)	375	?
Szarka (294)	363	?
Palik (253)	351	?
Lucisano (225)	345	?
Verrelli (310)	320	5.6
Lash (212)	313	–
Horvath (186)	310	?
Geneja et al. (174)[1]	299	–
Irmscher (187)	292	8.0
Zelkind and Djagilev (320)	265	–
Caresano (152)	261	–
Hilfrich et al. (180)	249	–
Kolos and Ferkó (207)	243	5.4
Mai (227)	235	9.2
Piechowiak et al. (256)	228	–
Archilei (129)	221	–
Krango et al. (209)	215	4.1
Hegyi and Radnoti (178)	212	?
Wittlinger (318)	212	11.8
Nobile et al. (246)	207	–
Loskant (224)	200	–

Table 3 (continued)

Author(s)	Cases	Proportion of all operations, %
Belopitov (138)	200	–
Dlhoš (165)	194	6.5
Mirkov and Atanasov (238)	180	–
Polito et al. (260)	168	13.4
Ahumada et al. (126)	165	7.6
Vácha and Stožický (307)	161	10.9
Camplani (151)	157	–
Stanca et al. (286)	155	–
Levinson and Potanova (218)	150	4.9
Fioretti and Andriani (171)	144	2.5
Boguňa et al. (144)	140	–
Trebicka (302)	124	3.8
Starostina (287)	122	–
Alicino and Pietrojusti (127)	120	4.4
Te Linde (299)	112	–
Zeman and Davids (321)	111	–
Bonanno (145)	109	14.0
Malato and Arienzo (228)	109	5.5
Mengaldo (235)	100	2.4
Gheorghiu and Iacob (175)[1]	100	–
Blanchard and Regueira (142)	87	–
Maurizio and Pescetto (231)	81	–
Károlyi (202)	76	9.5
Rio (268)	73	–
Danforth (161)	63	–
Lopatecki et al. (222)	60	–
Myasischev (243)	48	–
Total	29,691	–
Our material	6,658	

[1] From 61 years old onwards.

The overwhelming majority of the authors assumed an age limit of 60 years in the analysis of their operation material. The altered situation in our discipline is clearly shown in the fact that this age was still specified 20–30 years ago as the upper limit for general operability. In table 3 we have compiled the papers on women aged 60 or over. The proportion amongst all patients operated on was between 2.5 and 15.5%. The percentages depend on several factors – social structure of the population, time of evaluation, year of publication of the paper, etc.; no conclusions can thus be drawn from their differences.

Table 4. Studies on 65-year-old and older female patients

Author(s)	Cases	Proportion of all operations, %
Gause (173)	579	–
Muth (241)	512	5.3
Levy and Melchior (219)	476	–
Navratil (244)	474	–
Terzi et al. (300)	450	3.2
Paldi et al. (251)	239	–
Niesert and Seidenschnur (245)	227	6.8
McKeithen (234)	185	–
Krupa et al. (210)	181	–
Douglas (166)	163	–
Woraschk (319)	163	–
Douglas and Studdiford (167)	139	3.1
Decio (163)	139	–
Paldi et al. (252)	136	2.4
Tancer and Matseoane (297)	130	8.4
Sirtori (280)	129	–
Tancinco-Yambao and Lopez (298)	117	–
Piton (258)	110	–
Dalos (160)	105	?
Arenas and Bettinotti (132)	100	–
Bagnati and Villamayor (134)	92	–
Lefèvre (216)	65	–
Bourg and Piton (148)	40	–
Iwaszkiewicz (188)	34	2.7
Total	4,985	–
Our material	4,281	–

By far the largest number (5,615 cases) could be analyzed by *Vácha* (306). The patient material from 21 Czechoslovak gynecological departments was available to him. The largest body of data from one gynecological department (1,550 cases) was published by *Pernecker* (255). However, she used it almost exclusively for an exhaustive analysis of various methods of anesthesia. Then come papers by *Berle et al.* (141) with 1,514 cases, *Štefánik* (289) with 767 as well as *Bailo et al.* (135b) with 708 cases. The oldest paper by *Rusch* (271) with 496 large and 503 small gynecological interventions has never been cited in the literature so far. There is no doubt that in the future only studies with a similar order of size can contribute to solving the existing problems.

This also applies to the papers on 65-year-old and older operation patients (table 4). These also make up a considerable proportion of all operations, e.g. *Niesert and Seidenschnur* (245) 6.8%, *Muth* (241) 5.3%, *Tancer and Matseoane*

Table 5. Studies on 70-year-old and older female patients

Author(s)	Cases	Proportion of all operations, %
Rupprecht and Stange (270)	399	2.4
Braitenberg (149)	325	2.6
Lewis (220)	316	2.9
Widholm et al. (314)	309	1.0
Schürmann (276)	214	1.8
Macků and Kubečka (226)[1]	161	2.8
Dieminger (164)	142	2.3
Wendl (313)	129	2.9
Schilling and Schneck (274)	114	2.5
Carroll and Stoddard (153)	112	–
Bentzen and Anker (139)	100	–
Uhlmann (304)	73	?
Notelowicz (248)	50	–
Total	2,444	–
Our material	2,277	–

[1] From 71 years old onwards.

(297) 8.4%. With increasing expectation of life, this age will probably be regarded as the standard limit for surgical geriatric gynecology in the coming years.

As can be seen from table 5, some authors, e.g. *Skiftis et al.* (281) 3.7%, can show higher figures, even in 70-year-old and older patients. *Moustamindy* (240) has been the only author so far to have analyzed gynecological operations in patients over 75 years: 75–80 years, 44 women; 80–85 years, 19 women; 85–90 years, 5 women.

In our material, 261 women were at least 80 years old. Their operations have already been analyzed. Our communication (195) is only the second review after the paper by *Uzel and Kolářová* (305) which is exclusively concerned with operations in patients who are so old.

The oldest patients who have undergone operations reported in the literature are: 101 years old (135a), 95 years old (167), 91 years old (135a), 90 years old (242, 307), 89 years old (259), 87 years old (213), 86 years old (138, 228), 85 years old (226, 238, 297), 84 years old (246), and 82 years old (281, 305). Operations on very old women have also been reported in various casuistic contributions. For example, *Liccione* (221) reported on semicolpocleisis in a 96-year-old patient and *Jalůvka and Felshart* (356) described an operation of granulosa cell tumor in a 90-year-old woman.

Table 6. Studies with age groups at 5-year intervals in female patients at least 60 years old

Author(s)	Total cases	Age groups								
		60–64 years		65–69 years		70–74 years		75–79 years		80 years and over	
		cases	%	cases	%	cases	%	cases	%	cases	%
Alicino and Pietrojusti (127)[1]	120	67	55.8	32	26.3	14	11.6	6	5.0	1	0.8
Archilei (129)	221	89	40.2	66	29.8	43	19.4	16	7.2	7	3.1
Bailo et al. (135b)	708	411	58.6	198	28.2	72	10.3	20	2.8	1	0.1
Belopavlovič et al. (137)	545	258	47.3	174	31.9	77	14.1	32	5.9	4	0.8
Berger et al. (140)	682	304	44.7	222	32.8	112	16.5	35	5.1	7	0.9
Blobel and Häussler (143)[2]	366	152	41.5	135	36.9	59	16.1	15	4.1	5	1.4
Boguña et al. (144)	140	77	55.0	36	25.7	19	13.6	5	3.6	3	2.1
Caresano (152)	261	133	51.0	83	31.8	36	13.7	8	3.1	1	0.4
Fioretti and Andriani (171)	144	79	54.8	42	29.1	17	11.8	5	3.4	1	0.6
Geneja et al. (174)[2]	299	173	57.8	74	24.8	36	12.1	15	5.0	1	0.3
Lash (212)[1]	313	173	55.3	89	28.4	29	9.3	18	5.8	4	1.2
Levinson and Potanova (218)	150	55	36.7	42	28.0	22	14.7	20	13.3	11	7.3
Lucisano (225)	345	202	58.5	99	28.7	35	10.1	6	1.7	3	0.8
Malato and Arienzo (228)	109	60	55.1	25	22.9	18	16.5	6	5.5	–	–
Mengaldo (235)	100	62	62.0	23	23.0	11	11.0	4	4.0	–	–
Mirkov and Atanasov (238)[1]	180	121	67.2	42	23.4	10	5.6	4	2.2	3	1.6
Nobile et al. (246)[2]	207	102	49.3	70	33.8	25	12.1	10	4.8	–	–
Noci et al. (247)	34	20	58.9	9	26.4	4	11.8	1	2.9	–	–
Pernecker (255)	2,468	1,092	44.2	712	28.9	414	16.8	195	7.9	55	2.2
Piechowiak et al. (256)	228	116	50.9	60	26.3	32	14.0	17	7.5	3	1.3
Polito et al. (260)	168	77	46.0	50	29.7	32	19.0	7	4.1	2	1.2
Rieppi et al. (266)	532	257	48.3	180	33.8	75	14.1	18	3.4	2	0.4
Rigó and Zubek (267)	706	265	37.6	212	30.1	128	18.2	76	10.8	23	3.3
Rio (268)	73	34	46.6	18	24.6	14	19.2	3	4.1	4	5.5

Rusch (271)	496	276	55.6	149	30.0	54	10.9	17	3.5	—	—
Skiftis et al. (281)	398	172	43.2	112	28.2	76	19.1	38	9.5	—	—
Suonoja et al. (293)	573	261	45.5	183	31.9	92	16.1	24	4.2	13	2.3
Trebicka (302)	124	58	46.8	48	38.7	8	6.4	10	8.1	—	—
Trnka (303)	564	271	48.0	188	33.3	79	14.0	19	3.4	7	1.2
Verrelli (310)[2]	67	45	67.2	15	22.4	7	10.4	—	—	—	—

[1] 60—65 years, 66—70 years.
[2] 61—65 years.

Table 7. Studies with age groups at 5-year intervals in female patients at least 65 years old and in female patients at least 70 years old

Author(s)	Total cases	Age groups							
		65–69 years		70–74 years		75–79 years		80 years and over	
		cases	%	cases	%	cases	%	cases	%
Arenas and Bettinotti (132)[1]	100	70	70.0	16	16.0	12	12.0	2	2.0
Bagnati and Villamayor (134)[1]	92	66	71.7	20	21.7	4	4.4	2	2.2
Bulfoni et al. (150)	72	38	52.7	12	16.7	18	25.0	4	5.6
Curiel and Morresi (159)[1]	481	309	64.2	123	25.6	39	8.1	10	2.1
Decio (163)[1]	204	96	47.0	71	34.8	31	15.2	6	3.0
Douglas and Studdiford (167)	131	66	50.4	35	26.7	20	15.3	10	7.6
Krupa et al. (210)[2]	181	138	76.3	31	17.1	12	6.6	–	–
Levy and Melchior (219)	476	251	52.6	205	43.2	–	–	20	4.2
McKeithen (234)	185	67	36.2	58	31.4	49	26.5	11	5.9
Navratil (244)	474	227	47.9	172	36.3	64	13.5	11	2.3
Niesert and Seidenschnur (245)	227	133	58.6	66	29.1	20	8.8	8	3.5
O'Leary and Symmonds (250)	133	73	54.9	41	30.8	13	9.8	6	4.5
Paldi et al. (252)[1]	136	106	78.0	23	17.0	5	3.6	1	0.7
Sirtori (280)	129	89	69.0	32	24.8	7	5.4	1	0.8
Terzi et al. (300)[1]	614	406	66.0	144	23.5	48	8.0	16	2.5
Bentzen and Anker (139)[3]	100			43	43.0	40	40.0	17	17.0
Carroll and Stoddard (153)	112			74	66.1	31	27.7	7	6.2
Dieminger (164)	142			95	66.9	43	30.3	4	2.8
Lewis (220)	305			182	59.7	88	28.8	35	11.5
Mackù and Kubečka (226)[3]	161			114	70.8	36	22.4	11	6.8

[1] 65–70 years, 71–75 years.
[2] 66–70 years.
[3] 71–75 years.

Age Groups

The material was often divided into different age groups to enable a better overview. Tables 6 and 7 present the communications broken down into age groups at 5-year intervals. Attention is drawn in footnotes to individual differences. The age group '85 years old and over' was mentioned relatively rarely, so we included them in the age group '80–84 years old'. The greatest proportion of the operated patients was of course listed in the first two age groups. However, the absolute figures in higher age groups clearly show that large operations are also no longer an exception here. Table 8 is mainly intended to show the limited comparability of the age groups with a 10-year interval.

Table 8. Studies with age groups at 10-year intervals

Author(s)	Total cases	Age groups						Years		
		1st group		2nd group		3rd group		1st group	2nd group	3rd group
		cases	%	cases	%	cases	%			
Dlhoš (165)	194	143	73.7	50	25.8	1	0.5	60–70	71–80	80 and over
Horn et al. (184)	670	557	83.1	108	16.1	5	0.8	60–69	70–79	80 and over
Károlyi (202)	76	53	69.7	22	28.9	1	1.4	61–70	71–80	80 and over
Kolářová and Staníček (206)	375	255	68.1	100	26.6	20	5.3	60–70	70–80	80 and over
Krango et al. (209)	215	176	81.9	37	17.2	2	0.9	60–70	70–80	80 and over
Mai (227)	235	168	71.5	55	23.4	12	5.1	60–69	70–79	80 and over
Stanca et al. (286)	155	120	77.4	32	20.6	3	1.9	60–70	70–80	80 and over
Vácha (306)	5,615	4,078	74.9	1,242	22.8	125	2.3	60–69	70–79	80 and over
Muth (241)	213	153	72.0	58	27.0	2	1.0	65–70	71–80	81 and over
	299	163	54.0	122	41.0	14	5.0	66–75	75–85	86 and over
Tancinco-Yambao and Lopez (298)	117	92	78.6	18	15.4	7	6.0	61–70	71–80	–
Irmscher (187)	292	250	85.6	42	14.4	–	–	61–70	71–80	
Macků and Kubečka (226)	161	150	93.2	11	6.8	–	–	60–69	70 and over	
Maurizio and Pescetto (231)	81	68	84.0	13	16.0	–	–	61–69	70 and over	
Wittlinger (318)	212	111	52.1	101	47.9	–	–	60–69	70 and over	
Piton (258)	110	80	72.7	30	27.3	–	–	60–69	70 and over	
Randow and Riess (263)	633	475	75.0	158	25.0	–	–	65–75	76 and over	
Starostina (287)	122	107	87.7	15	12.3	–	–	61–70	71–83	
Vácha and Stožický (307)	161	119	73.9	42	26.1	–	–	60–69	70–82	

Table 9. Increase of geriatric patients in the total operation material

Author(s)	Age	Proportion of geriatric patients in total operation material	
		years	%
Berle et al. (141)	60	1947–1959	9.8
		1960–1972	16.9
Bailo et al. (135b)	60	1951–1955	6.4
		1956–1960	8.2
		1961–1965	9.7
Vácha (306)	60	1959	12.6
		1960	13.0
		1961	12.7
		1962	13.8
		1963	14.3
Muth (241)	65	1925–1931	1.0
		1932–1937	1.6
		1938–1943	2.1
		1944–1949	2.3
		1950–1955	4.3
		1956–1961	5.2
Niesert and Seidenschnur (245)	65	1935–1939	1.6
		1952–1957	6.8
Braitenberg (149)	70	1936–1940	1.1
		1956–1960	3.6
Dieminger (164)	70	1951–1955	1.2
		1956–1963	2.3 Irmscher (187)
Schürmann (276)	70	1940–1944	0.7
		1945–1949	0.9
		1950–1954	2.0
		1955–1959	2.6
		1960–1963	4.2
Widholm et al. (314)	70	1951–1956	0.7
		1957–1961	1.4
Wendl (313)	70	1942–1947	0.2
		1948–1953	0.5
		1954–1959	2.9

Increase of Geriatric Patients in the Operation Material

Table 9 informs on the increase in the surgical geriatric patient material. This is to be explained by two factors: more women reach the corresponding age, and there is an intensive and successful cooperation with other specialist disciplines. The former leads to an absolute increase in the proportion of geriatric operations in the total gynecological operation material, and the latter to a relative increase.

Concomitant Diseases

By the somewhat arbitrary fixing of 'the age limit' at 60 years, little consideration is given to the individual course of biological aging. There is an immense literature on its general (basically physiological) processes and on numerous chronic conditions of elderly women. We should therefore like to restrict ourselves in this connection to the analysis of the studies which have already been mentioned.

The data in table 10 are only partly comparable. This is due among other factors to the non-uniform designation of the clinical picture and the differing thoroughness of the analysis of material. This is confirmed indirectly by *Vácha* (306) in the analysis of material deriving from 21 hospitals, when he does not mention concomitant diseases at all. Only *Zeman and Davids* (321) as well as *Niesert and Seidenschnur* (245) have classified the concomitant diseases according to single organs. In this way, the rare but nonetheless significant complications can better be taken into account.

All analyses indicate that cardiovascular complications are the most frequent in geriatric gynecological operations. *Starostina* (288) treats this problem in a communication devoted specifically to it. It would be of clinical value to set up a larger comparison collective to investigate cardiovascular complications.

The lower limit of hypertension (systolic blood pressure) has for instance been specified at quite different levels: *Horn et al.* (185) 170–200 and over 200 mm Hg; *Lash* (212) 170 mm Hg; *Lucisano* (225) 165–200 and over 200 mm Hg; *Muth* (241) 180 mm Hg; *Piton* (258) 160 mm Hg; *Randow and Riess* (263) 180 mm Hg; *Rigó and Zubek* (267) 160–200 and over 200 mm Hg; *Stanca et al.* (286) 200 mm Hg. *Curiel and Morresi* (159), *Rio* (268) as well as *Polito et al.* (260) have undertaken an analysis of blood pressure values at intervals of 10 mm Hg. For *Lewis* (220), only the diastolic values were decisive. In 70 out of 305 patients, they were over 100 mm Hg.

Varicosis has been specified in only a few papers and with considerably varying proportions: *Randow and Riess* (263) 55%, *Muth* (241) 45.3%, *Stanca et al.* (286) 9.7% as well as *Piton* (258) 2.7%. The frequent lack of any data on

Table 10. Accompanying diseases in operated geriatric-gynecological patients

Author(s)	Cases	Accompanying diseases
Ahumada et al. (126)	165	hypertension 54.5%, diabetes 9%, cardiopathy 6.6%, liver diseases 5.4%, obesity 4.8%, varices 4.8%, lung diseases 3.6%
Alicino and Pietrojusti (127)	120	hypertension over 170 mm Hg 26, anemia 9, diabetes 9, cardiopathy 5, hepatopathy 5
Archilei (129)	221	cardiovascular diseases 15, varices 9, hypertension over 160 mm Hg 8, chronic bronchitis 8, bronchial asthma 6
Ardelt et al. (131)	660	ECG pathological in 63.6% (slight in 37.8%, marked in 25.8%), hypertension 50.6% (160/95 26.7%, 180/100 17.7%, 200/120 6.2%), aortic sclerosis (chest X-ray) 46.7%, obesity (80 kg) 12.7%, diabetes mellitus 11.5% (diet and tablets 9.7%, insulin-dependent 1.8%), Quick 70% 7.7%, anemia (Hb 60%) 1.2%, without pathological finding 3.6%
Bagnati and Villamayor (134)	92	hypertension 12, diabetes 5, anemia 3, etc.
Bailo et al. (135b)	708	hypertension and arteriosclerosis 305, arrhythmias 18, relative circulatory decompensation 14, myocardial infarction 19, slight renal insufficiency 26, chronic bronchitis and asthma 53, diabetes 27, anemia 6
Berger et al. (140)	681	'cardiovascular' complications 211, hypertension 88, respiratory complications 23, diabetes 18, urological complications 15, anemia 9
Boguňa et al. (144)	190 (140)	obesity 14, anemia 12, varices 12, malnutrition 10, etc.
Bulfoni et al. (150)	72	hypertension 24, ischemic cardiopathy 11, adiposity 16
Carroll and Stoddard (153)	112	arteriosclerotic heart diseases 13, angina pectoris 3, arrhythmias 3, coronary symptoms 2, cardiac decompensation 2, diabetes 4
Dlhoš (165)	194	normal internal finding 45, hypertension 51, heart disease 36, arteriosclerosis 34, other diseases 28
Douglas and Studdiford (167)	131	essential hypertension 43, hypertensive cardiovascular disease 36, obesity 28, arteriosclerotic cardiovascular disease 22, generalized arteriosclerosis 10, diabetes 9, arthritis 5, pulmonary emphysema 4
Fioretti and Andriani (171)	144	hypertension 51, cardiovascular diseases 50, varices 20, etc.
Károlyi (202)	76	cardiovascular pathology 27.6%, pulmonary pathology 19.7%, hypertension (?) 60.6% and over 200 mm Hg 15.2%

Table 10 (continued)

Author(s)	Cases	Accompanying diseases
Lash (212)	313	hypertension over 140 mm Hg 217, hypertension over 170 mm Hg 111, diabetes 12, hemiplegia 7, asthma 5, arthritis 4, psychosis 1
Lewis (220)	305	anemia 27 (Hb under 80%), heart defect 30, diabetes 10, diastolic blood pressure over 100 mm Hg 70
Lucisano (225)	345	hypertension 165–200 mm Hg 134 (38.8%), over 200 mm Hg 40 (11.6%), disease of the cardiovascular system 184 (52.8%), obesity 60, emphysema 17, chronic bronchitis 11, etc.
Malato and Arienzo (228)	109	respiratory complications 5, cardiac complications 17, circulatory complications 32, metabolic complications 9, other complications 7
Mengaldo (235)	100	hypertension 31, anemia 12, chronic bronchitis 8, varices 17, hepatopathy 11, etc.
Muth (241)	299	pathological ECG finding 151 (50.6%), varicosis 136 (45.3%), hypertension 180 mm Hg and more 81 (27%), obesity 44 (13%), diabetes 22 (7%), anemia 21 (6.8%), cachexia 19 (6.3%), emphysema 11 (3.6%)
Niesert and Seidenschnur (245)	227	cardiovascular system: myocardial damage 90, hypertension 65, defects 2, coronary insufficiency 6; metabolic disorders: obesity over 85 kg, malnutrition; cachexia 35, disturbed water balance 23, biliary tract infection 2; respiratory tract: severe emphysemal bronchitis 29; hematopoietic system: anemia 19
O'Leary and Symmonds (250)	133	hypertension 78, heart diseases 48, obesity 46, chronic lung diseases 8, anemia 8, diabetes 8
Paldi et al. (251)	239	hypertension 85, arteriosclerosis 31, rheumatic heart disease 8, diabetes 17, asthma 6, cholelithiasis 12, obesity 12, etc.
Piechowiak et al. (256)	228	hypertension 122, anemia 32, cardiac insufficiency 10, diabetes 5
Piton (258)	110	cardiac affection 39, arteriosclerosis 54, hypertension over 160 mm Hg 49, respiratory affections 23, diabetes 12, varices 3
Polito et al. (260)	168	respiratory complications 35, cardiovascular complications 34, urological complications 6, diabetes 13, other pathology 32
Randow and Riess (263)	633	hypertension over 180 mm Hg 314 (50%), degenerative and hypoxic myocardial damage 368 (58%), varicosis 348 (55%), pulmonary diseases 150 (23%), diabetes 18 (3%)

Table 10 (continued)

Author(s)	Cases	Accompanying diseases
Rieppi et al. (266)	532	cardiopathy 291 (54.7%), hypertension 244 (45.9%), emphysema 271 (50.9%), other complications 123 (23.1%)
Rigó and Zubek (267)	704	internal diseases: cardiovascular diseases 123 (17.4%), gastrointestinal diseases 61 (8.6%), diabetes 46 (6.5%), arthritis 39 (5.5%), jaundice 36 (5.1%), pulmonary tuberculosis 25 (3.4%), hypertension 160–200 mm Hg 305 (43.2%), over 200 mm Hg 76 (10.2%)
Stanca et al. (286)	155	cardiopathy 28, hypertension over 200 mm Hg 40, chronic bronchitis 12, varices 15, diabetes 7, etc.
Štefánik (289)	367	hypertension 137, cardiosclerosis 89, varicosis 44, diseases of the respiratory tract, diseases of the gastrointestinal tract, defects 39, other diseases 21
Suonoja et al. (293)	573	hypertension 140 (24.4%), cardiac decompensation and coronary insufficiency 114 (19.9%), diabetes mellitus 30 (5.2%), diseases of the respiratory tract 21 (3.7%), varices 19 (3.3%)
Trebicka (302)	124	chronic myocarditis 10, hypertension 7, cachexia 6, chronic bronchitis 1, emphysema 2
Vácha and Stožický (307)	161	pulmonary emphysema and chronic bronchitis 67 (37.9%), hypertension and arteriosclerosis and ischemic heart diseases 106 (65.8%), diabetes 5 (3.1%), obesity 58 (36.6%), cachexia 5 (3.1%)
Wittlinger (317)	212	hypertension over 160/100 mm Hg 44.7%, cardiac insufficiency (digitalis required) 19.3%, myocardial damage in the ECG 16.0%, chronic bronchitis, emphysema 23.6%, moderate obesity (20–30 kg over the ideal weight) 15.6%, severe obesity (more than 30 kg) 22.6%, marked varicosity 15.7%, diabetes mellitus 11.3%, rise in urea over 50 mg% 4.6%
Zeman and Davids (321)	202	cardiovascular system (139): rheumatic diseases 60, arteriosclerosis 57, metabolic disorders (56): obesity 20, poor nutrition 26, diabetes 10, hematopoietic system (34): anemia 32, respiratory system 3, urogenital system 5

varicosis indicates that many authors have regarded it as a complication which was not worth mentioning. Anemia is often present among the concomitant diseases. We have always failed to see any note as to what preoperative treatment had been given to the existing anemia. Unfortunately, corresponding laboratory values were practically always lacking. The following studies constitute an exception. In the operation material of *Curiel and Morresi* (159), the following hemoglobin values had been determined before the operation: $\leqslant 10.0$ g in 10 women (3%), $10.1-12$ g in 51 women (15.5%), $12-14$ g in 138 women (41.8%) and $\geqslant 14.1$ g in 131 women (39.7%). *Lewis* (220) found a hemoglobin value under 80% in 27 out of 306 patients; 6 women received a blood transfusion before the intervention.

We found two further sets of data on the blood picture in *Polito et al.* (260): 8 g hemoglobin in 5 women (2.9%), $8.1-10$ g in 16 women (9.5%), $10.1-12$ g in 120 women (71.4%), $12.1-14$ g in 27 women (16.0%). 6 women (3.5%) had less than 3 million erythrocytes, 29 (17.2%) had $3-3.5$ million, 96 (57.1%) had $3.5-4.0$ million and 35 (20.8%) had $4.0-4.5$ million erythrocytes. According to *Torsello and Palazzetti* (301), the reduced blood volume and the hypoproteinemia are to be regarded as aging phenomena. On the other hand, the other hematological data may have a pathological significance.

The study by *Rieppi et al.* (266) is a valuable contribution to the problem of concomitant diseases. These authors have not only listed the individual diseases, but have analyzed the simultaneous occurrence of hypertension, other alterations of the cardiovascular system and pulmonary emphysema. They have thus clearly pointed out the existence of multimorbidity in elderly and aged women. Some authors have undertaken a combined analysis of concomitant diseases in individual age groups or in vaginal and abdominal interventions (155, 159, 245, 257, 261, 318).

Nutritional State

A significant preoperative factor is the nutritional state. This is mostly taken into account with data on the frequency of obesity (table 10). On the other hand, there have only rarely been reports on the frequency of malnutrition or cachexia due to tumors. Sometimes one finds a general note on disturbances of serum protein balance and a shift in the water and electrolyte balance.

Assessment of the Risk of Operation

For objectivation of the surgical risk, *Loskant* (224) divided his patients into four risk groups and has thus shown a way for better assessment of the surgical prognosis (table 11). His observation that in recent years there has been

Table 11. Scheme of operative risks after *Loskant* (224)

	Risk group I (without foreseeable risk)	Risk group II (slight impairment of organ and system functions)	Risk group III (raised risk)	Risk group IV (highly raised risk)
Cases	20 (10.0%)	76 (38.0%)	71 (35.5%)	33 (16.5%)
General condition (clinical impression)	good	moderate	reduced	poor
Lungs	without symptoms or findings	e.g. slight ('senile') emphysema, condition after lung infections, etc.	e.g. pulmonary emphysema, extensive adhesive pleurisy, (asthmoid) bronchitis, bronchial asthma, etc.	e.g. severe emphysema, pneumonia, pleural effusion, severe asthma, pneumothorax, etc.
Heart	without symptoms or findings	e.g. incipient diminution of cardiac performance, ECG alterations without symptoms, etc.	e.g. latent cardiac insufficiency, angina pectoris, ECG alterations with symptoms (conduction disturbance), etc.	e.g. cardiac insufficiency, absolute arrhythmia, partial or total block, condition after infarction, etc.
Circulation	without symptoms or findings	e.g. demonstrable arteriosclerosis without appreciable symptoms, hypertension, disturbance of orthostatic regulation, etc.	e.g. arteriosclerosis with disturbance of vascular function and blood distribution, severe hypertension, etc.	severe hypertension with signs of cardiac decompensation, postapoplectic states, severe cerebral sclerosis, etc.
Diabetes	without symptoms or findings	e.g. slight ('senile') diabetes with diabetic stabilization and therapy, etc.	e.g. diabetes with tendency to lapses and specific organ changes (vessels), etc.	e.g. acidosis, prediabetic coma, severe organ damage (diabetic gangrene), etc.

Danger of thrombosis	without symptoms or findings	e.g. isolated varices	e.g. varicosis, adiposity	e.g. severe varicosis, extensive thrombophlebitis, anamnestic thromboses and embolism, etc.
Other	without symptoms or findings	no prospective influence on course of operation or anesthesia, e.g. anemia up to Hb 10 g%, glaucoma, etc.	prospective influence on course of operation or anesthesia: e.g. kidney damage disturbance of electrolyte and water balance, slight liver damage, hyperthyroidism, fever, tracheomalacia, etc.	prospective severe influence on course of operation or anesthesia; e.g. jaundice, adrenal cortical insufficiency, ileus, etc.

Table 12. Scheme of risks after *Loskant* (224) and the selective classification criteria (180)

Risk group	Criteria
I	ϕ
II	pulmonary emphysema slight hypertension RR 160/95 to 180/100 mm Hg
III	latent cardiac insufficiency slight cardiac insufficiency and/or hypertension 180/100 mm Hg and/or coronary insufficiency
IV	manifest cardiac insufficiency and/or ventricular insufficiency, cor pulmonale and/or cardiac asthma and/or status asthmaticus and/or insulin-dependent diabetes mellitus and/or anemia Hb 50% and/or adipositas permagna in abdominal operations and/or chronic bronchitis

a marked increase in the frequency of operations in the groups with raised and greatly raised risk is important. His classification has in the meantime been employed by the following authors: *Schilling and Schneck* (274) assigned from their 114 patients 17.5% of the women to the first risk group, 28% to the second risk group, 30.8% to the third risk group and 23.7% to the fourth risk group. *Berger et al.* (140) assigned to the first risk group 308 patients (44.7%), to the second risk group 149 (21.9%), to the third risk group 204 (29.9%) and to the fourth risk group 20 (3.5%). *Wittlinger* (317) assigned to the first risk group 31 patients (14.6%), to the second risk group 44 (20.8%), to the third risk group 90 (42.5%) and to the fourth risk group 47 (22.1%).

The *Barth and Meyer* (136b) classification of the surgical risk is qualitatively the same as that used by *Muth* (241). According to *Muth*, the patients are also mainly assigned to group two and three: first risk group (no organ or systemic injuries) 16 patients (5.4%), second risk group (slight to moderate organ or systemic damage) 157 (52.4%), third risk group (severe organ or systemic damage) 98 (32.8%), fourth risk group (very severe organ or systemic damage) 28 (9.4%).

Polito et al. (260) evaluate the state of cardiovascular, respiratory and uropoietic systems at three levels: 'superiore alla norma con (+), di discreta gravita con (++), di notevole gravita con (+++)'. *Curiel and Morresi* (159) have proceeded similarly in renal, cardiovascular and general diseases. We failed to

Table 13. Modified scheme on the risk of surgery according to *Göltner* (see 180)

Points	Duration of operation, min	Infusion, ml
0	0–50	0–500
1	50–100	500–1,000
2	100–150	1,000–1,500
3	150–200	1,500–2,000
4	200 and over	2,000 and over

find data on objective characteristics in both communications. *Rio* (268) divided his patients into three groups: '(1) superiore alla norma, (2) medio, (3) elaborato'. *Noci et al.* (247) classified the risk in their operated patients into four groups: 'normale, superiore alla norma (+), di media gravita (++), di notevole grado (+++)'.

Stožický and Vácha (291) formed three risk groups: (1) patients with internal findings corresponding to their age; (2) patients with pathological findings which raised the surgical risk but which were not a contraindication to intervention, and (3) patients with grave internal complications, but also with vital indications for gynecological intervention.

The schematic nature of the suggestions cannot be overlooked, and objective criteria are lacking in almost all. The subjective assessment substantially restricts the usefulness of these risk schemata.

Hilfrich et al. (180) went a step further with the allocation of different internal diseases into the schemes specified by *Loskant* (224) (table 12). As expected, they were able to detect postoperatively a direct correlation between the number of complications which had occurred and the individual groups. The frequent application of such preoperative schemata, most satisfactorily with inclusion also of the complications of other organs and systems, would be desirable.

Consideration of the surgery risk is also a positive contribution by *Hilfrich et al.* (180) (table 13). With increasing degree of risk, they were able to demonstrate an increasing frequency of (especially of severe) postoperative complications. The risk scheme can of course not be applied before the planned intervention. This does not diminish its usefulness, since today it is less the operations themselves than the postoperative complications which constitute a danger for the patient. *Hilfrich et al.* have correlated both the risk of operation as well as surgical stress simultaneously with the postoperative complications which arose. With increase of the two parameters, the complications also increased markedly. The view of the author that the procedures he applied

Table 14. Evaluation of the risk of surgery according to *Henriquet* (179)

	Points
Age	
Under 60 years	1
Over 60 years	0
Weight	
Less than 15 kg over ideal weight	1
More than 15 kg over ideal weight	0
General conditions	
No organic diseases	3
No serious organic diseases	2
Severe organic diseases	0
Kind of operation	
Small interventions	4
Medium interventions	3
Radical interventions	1
Eviscerations	0

Table 15. Risk diagnosis and assessment as prerequisite for prevention of intraoperative and postoperative complications (146)

I Diagnosis of the risks

Unavoidable risks
  From the disease
  From the condition of the patient
  From the planned intervention
    ↓
  Choice of preoperative diagnostic

Avoidable risks
  From surgical possibilities
  From instrumental possibilities
  From nursing possibilities
    ↓
  Choice of hospital

II Assessment of the risks

Vital indication for surgery (high risks are lower than the risks of surgery)
Indication for surgery (risks are to be weighed against the benefit of operation)
Operation when requested by the patient (even slight risks are higher than the benefit of the operation)

III Prevention of the risks

  Avoidance of operations entailing too high a risk
  Preventive therapy

enable a reliable prospective assessment of the postoperative course is to be affirmed.

Henriquet (179) has attempted to carry out a combined analysis of the risk of surgery taking into account the age, the weight, the general condition and the kind of operation. It is seen from table 14 that in the optimum case, a young, healthy woman could receive 9 points. The lower the number of points, the greater the risk of surgery. The figures of *Henriquet* can only partly be applied to our problem, since he considered all patients (i.e. also those younger than 60 years old) and all interventions. The 1,067 patients who were operated on in his patient material had the following degree of operability expressed in points: 160 women (15.0%) had 9 points; 348 (32.6%) had 8 points; 293 (27.5%) had 7 points; 123 (11.5%) had 6 points; 83 (7.8%) had 5 points; 32 (3.0%) had 4 points, and 28 (2.6%) had 3 points.

The applicability of such risk schemata should not only be checked on the total operation material, but also separately for diseases with relative and absolute or vital indication for surgery. *Börner* (146) does not content himself with diagnosis of the risks, but also considers them carefully and suggests their prevention (table 15).

In the preoperative assessment of the state of health of the patients, the capacity to undergo anesthesia must be taken into account besides the general operability. Only in this way can the specific concerns of the anesthetist be given sufficient weight. A further intensification of the cooperation between the surgical disciplines and the internists and anesthetists interested in general geriatric problems could best contribute to qualitative improvement of preoperative examination and assessment of the risk of surgery. A good example here is the checklist for risk classification by *Lutz et al.* (cited in 146) (table 16).

We found the clinically important note of the number of operations which, although indicated, were not carried out because of the great risk, only in the following studies: *Rio* (268) operated on only 73 women out of 90 admitted for surgery. *Arenas and Bettinotti* (132) found a contraindication to surgical treatment 24 times among 124 women admitted. *Mirkov and Atanasov* (238) reported on 225 women admitted for operation (60–90 years old): in 8 cases the descensus was treated conservatively, in 16 it was an inoperable carcinoma, 17 had cardiovascular decompensation and 4 had refused the suggested operation. The foreseen surgical intervention was thus carried out in 180 women. *Malato and Arienzo* (228) gave less detailed data: of the 154 women admitted, 109 were operated on. Similarly, *Polito et al.* (260) record 231 patients admitted and 168 operated on.

It would also be very important to learn more about the number of cases declared to be inoperable in the outpatients department (malignancies) and especially about the genital displacements. However, we have been totally unable to find corresponding data in the literature.

Table 16. Checklist for risk classification in the form worked out by *Lutz et al.* with modifications brought about by long use in surgical gynecology (see 146)

	Points					
	0	1	2	4	8	15
Treatment	inpatients	outpatients	emergency admission			
Operation	plan	urgent	emergency admission			
Age	3–39	40–69	70–79	up to 3/from 80		
Weight	normal + 10%	+ 10–30% − 10–15%	+ 30–50% − 15–25%	>50% >25%		
Last meal	>6h	<6 h	<3 h	<1 h		
Conscious-ness	clear	drugs	convulsive attacks in anamnesis	clouded	comatose	
Circulation	stable	hypotension	labile hypertension	fixed hypertension	compens. shock	decompens. shock
Heart function	healthy	organic heart defect fully compensated	fall in performance in exercise	infarct more than 3 months previously	compens. cardiac insuff.	decompens. cardiac insuff.
Digitali-zation	digitalized	non-digitalized				
Cardiac rhythm	normal	disturbed	AV block III	tachyar-rhythmia absoluta	ventricular extrasystoles	
Respiration	normal vital capacity 80%	impaired vital capacity 70%	broncho-pulmonary disease vital capacity 60–70%	pneumonia vital capacity 50–60%	vital capacity 50%	
Kidney function	normal	renal insuff. creat. clear. <80 ml/min	renal insuff. creat. clear. <50 ml/min	anuria creat. clear. <30 ml/min	uremia	
Liver function	normal	bilirubin in serum 20 μmol/l CHE 1,900 U/l	bilirubin >40 μmol/l CHE < 1,000 U/L	bilirubin >70 μmol/l CHE < 800 U/l	hepatic coma	

Table 16 (continued)

	Points					
	0	1	2	4	8	15
Sugar metabolism	normal	orally comp. senile diabetes	insulin-requiring diabetes	diabetes which is difficult to compensate		
Electro-lytes	normal	$K^+ > 5$ mV/l $Na^+ > 15$ mV/l	$K^+ < 3$ mV/l	$K^+ < 2.5$ mV/l		
Water balance	normal	hematocrit >40, osmol. <280 mosm/kg	hematocrit >50, total protein lowered	dehydration		
Hemoglobin	>12.5 g%	12.5–7.5 g%	<7.5 g%			
Prior operation	none	taxing prior operation				
Prospective duration of operation	<120 min	120–180 min	>180 min			

Risk levels: I = 0–1 points, II = 2–3 points, III = 4–7 points, IV = 8–15 points, V = ≥ 15 points.

Operation Material

The studies we have cited are almost exclusively concerned with the 'large' gynecological interventions. In almost all cases, the majority of authors leaves out the abrasions, radium depositions, exploratory excisions, conizations, and polyp removals. *Randow and Riess* (263) even account Labhardt, Kahr, Conill as well as Neugebauer-LeFort operations as being 'small' or 'miscellaneous' inter-ventions. All operations were analyzed in only a few studies (144, 184, 240, 255, 267, 271, 296, 297, 305, 321). We allowed ourselves to be guided by the literature and only analyzed 'large' operations. We should like to observe in retrospect that all interventions from sufficiently large operation material should be recorded under the term 'surgical geriatric gynecology'. The classification into 'small' and 'large' operations, which is not always easy, can be carried out retrospectively. Especially in the future, we should be more often concerned with special part problems of surgical geriatric gynecology (150, 159, 191–194, 196–200, 232, 247, 250, 257, 322).

Symptoms

Some authors have analyzed the clinical symptoms of women who were operated on (144, 167, 252, 268, 321). The value of these data is for our purposes slight because of the simultaneous analysis of disease symptoms which only required a small intervention. A compilation of the symptoms which led to admission would be useful. There have been no publications so far on these problems. We have also failed to find any data on the modalities of admission (family doctor, gynecologist, cancer prevention, random finding without symptoms etc.).

Table 17. Duration of treatment of geriatric gynecological patients

Author(s)	Age, years	Duration of treatment, days		
		total	before operation	after operation
Alicino and Pietrojusti (127)	60	31.2	13.0	18.2
Berle et al. (141)	60	40.3[1]	11.1	29.2
		31.6[2]	8.8	22.8
Dieminger (164)	70	32.0	11.0	21.0
Fioretti and Andriani (171)	60	33.4[1]	15.0	18.4
		31.6[2]	12.2	19.4
Rieppi et al. (266)	70	20.0	8.0	12.0
Schilling and Schneck (274)	70	36.2	?	?
Sirtori (280)	65	22.2[2]	8.6	13.6
		17.0[2]	5.3	11.7
		36.0[3]	9.6	26.4
Stanca et al. (286)	60	22.6	10.2	12.4
Szendi and Lakatos (296)	60	16—22	?	?
Wittlinger (317)	61	26.7 (?)	5.9	19.8

[1] Laparotomies.
[2] Vaginal operations.
[3] Vulvar operations.

Duration of Treatment

The duration of hospitalization before the operation does not only depend on the general state of health of the patient. For example, this time can be somewhat shortened by carrying out preoperative examinations as an outpatient. Even with smaller interventions and in women who had prior examinations, it is not advisable to aim for immediate operation when the patient is very old. It is known that precisely these patients frequently require a certain time for adaptation. This problem has already been dealt with in detail by *Cséffalvay et al.* (158).

Niesert and Seidenschnur (245) observed the following periods of preparation in their 227 70-year-old patients who were operated on: 1–2 days for 30 women, 3–4 days for 48, 5–7 days for 73, and more than 8 days for 76. *Piton* (258) contented himself with the observation that the hospital stay of his 100 patients was more than 1 month on the average, with 15–20 days serving for preoperative preparation. According to *Lewis* (220) the inpatient stay of the 70-year-old and older patients averaged 21 days (6–67 days) and according to *Károlyi* (202) it was on the average 21.8 days (before the operation 8.2 and after the operation 13.6 days). *Károlyi* reported a difference between the 61- to 70-year-old patients (19 days) and the 71- to 84-year-old patients (26.6 days). The difference of 7.6 days is to be explained by the longer preoperative (4.7 days) and postoperative (2.9 days) inpatient stay in the older group. *Curiel and Morresi* (159) undertook the evaluation of the duration of inpatient treatment in 5-year age groups. Their relatively short inpatient stay (8.5 days before and 12.1 days after the operation) can be explained by the qualitative difference in their material (only benign pathology). In the patients of *Bonanno* (145) the inpatient stay lasted on average 13 days. *Blanchard and Regueira* (142) recorded the following treatment times in their patients: 1–10 days for 9 women, 11–20 days for 41, 21–30 days for 37, 31–40 days for 15, 41–50 days for 11, and more than 50 days for 7. Further data on the average duration of the preoperative and postoperative phases are to be found in table 17.

Anesthesia

Many authors have been concerned with this problem (126, 128, 130, 132, 134, 142, 145, 153, 162, 164, 167, 171, 173–176, 184, 202, 203, 205, 206, 218, 220, 225, 226, 233, 239, 245, 255, 266, 276, 313, 314, 320, 321). The diversity of the literature data makes it difficult to carry out a comprehensive comparison. Due to the rapid development of anesthesiology, other methods of anesthesia are found in the studies described 30 years ago (e.g. 212) than in modern studies (e.g. 241). The development of anesthesia is to be discerned especially clearly in the communications concerned with analysis of treatment over a longer period – *Schürmann* (276): 1930–1962 or *Štefánik* (289): 1933–1964.

Table 18. Indication for operation in studies on 60-year-old female patients

Author(s)	Total cases	Malignant tumors		Benign tumors		Genital displacements		Other	
		n	%	n	%	n	%	n	%
Ahumada et al. (126)	165	88	53.4	15	9.0	62	37.6	–	–
Ardelt et al. (131)	660	278	42.1	147	22.3	211	31.9	24	3.7
Bailo et al. (135b)	676	197	29.1	90	13.3	361	53.5	28	4.1
Berger et al. (140)	681	307	45.0	134	19.7	236	34.7	4	0.6
Boguňa et al. (144)	140	37	26.4	6	4.3	97	69.3	–	–
Camplani (151)	157	16	10.2	24	15.3	110	69.8	7	4.7
Fioretti and Andriani (171)	144	25	17.4	11	7.6	95	66.0	13	9.0
Hilfrich et al. (180)	249	117	46.9	42	16.9	79	31.8	11	4.4
Kolářová and Staníček (206)	375	170	45.3	30	8.0	135	36.0	40	10.7
Kolos and Ferkó (207)	243	87	35.8	42	17.3	111	45.7	3	1.2
Krango et al. (209)	215	38	17.7	30	14.0	137	63.7	10	4.6
Lucisano (225)	345	103	29.8	45[1]	13.2	167	48.3	30	8.7
Mai (227)	248	62	25.0	66	26.6	96	38.8	24	9.6
Malato and Arienzo (228)	109	28	25.7	37	34.0	38	34.8	6	5.5
Mengaldo (235)	100	9	9.0	11	11.0	75	75.0	5	5.0
Pernecker (255)	1,550	769	49.4	190	12.3	513	32.1	78	6.2
Polito et al. (260)	168	41	24.4	3	1.8	98	58.3	26	15.5
Rieppi et al. (266)	532	71	13.5	45	8.5	412	77.3	4	0.7
Rio (268)	73	7	9.6	9	12.4	45	61.6	12	16.4
Rusch (271)	497	223	45.0	70	14.0	184	37.0	20	4.0
Siliquini and Petterino (279)	633	102	16.1	154	24.3	209	34.7	168	24.9
Skiftis et al. (281)	398	154	38.7	75	18.8	136	34.2	33[2]	8.3
Stanca et al. (286)	155	32	20.6	8	9.2	95	61.3	20	12.9
Štefánik (289)	767	168	22.0	114	14.9	485	63.1	–	–
Suonoja et al. (293)	573	98	17.1	78	13.6	367	64.1	30	5.2
Trebicka (302)	124	22	17.8	23	18.6	77	62.0	2	1.6
Verrelli (311)	320	66	20.6	39	12.2	197	61.6	18	5.6
Wittlinger (317)	212	46	21.8	43	20.3	114	53.7	9	4.2
Zelkind and Djagilev (320)	265	59	22.3	130	49.0	71	26.8	5	1.9
Total	10,774	3,420	31.7	1,711	15.9	5,013	46.6	630	5.8

[1] Only uterine tumors.
[2] Emergencies.

Table 19. Indication for operation in studies of 65- to 70-year-old and older patients

Author(s)	Total cases	Malignant tumors		Benign tumors		Genital displacements		Other diseases	
		n	%	n	%	n	%	n	%
Arenas and Bettinotti (132)	100	37	37.0	8	8.0	47	47.0	8	8.0
Bagnati and Villamayor (134)	92	21	22.8	12	13.2	54	58.6	5	5.4
Bourg and Piton (148)	40	13	32.5	3	7.5	24	60.0	–	–
Curiel and Morresi (159)	481	–	–	49	10.4	388	80.5	44	9.1
Decio (163)	139	61	44.0	11	7.9	66	47.4	1	0.7
Iwaszkiewicz (188)	34	8	23.6	2	5.9	24	70.5	–	–
Krupa et al. (210)	181	58	32.0	?	?	105	58.0	18	10.0
Navratil (244)	474	194	41.0	95	20.0	162	34.2	23	4.8
Niesert and Seidenschnur (245)	227	86	38.0	24	10.6	106	46.6	11	4.8
Paldi et al. (251)	239	46	19.3	28	11.7	156	65.3	9	3.7
Piton (258)	110	31	28.2	13	11.8	53	48.2	13	11.8
Sirtori (280)	129	31	24.0	11	8.5	83	64.4	4	3.1
Tancinco-Yambao and Lopez (298)	99	5	5.1	17	17.2	63	63.6	14	14.1
Terzi et al. (300)	484	219	54.0	73	18.0	192	28.0	–	–
Woraschk (319)	163	75	46.0	30	18.4	49	30.1	9	5.5
Total	2,992	885	29.5	376	12.6	1,572	52.6	159	5.3
Bentzen and Anker (139)	99	20	20.0	5	5.0	68	69.0	6	6.0
Carroll and Stoddard (153)	112	18	16.0	3	2.7	91	81.3	0	0
Lewis (220)	305	86	28.2	29	9.5	190	62.3	–	–
Macků and Kubečka (226)	161	41	25.5	30	18.6	90	55.9	–	–
Rupprecht and Stange (270)	399	157	39.3	56	14.2	177	44.3	9	2.2
Schilling and Schneck (274)	114	51	44.7	27	23.7	34	29.8	2	1.8
Widholm et al. (314)	309	82	26.5	71	23.0	134	43.3	22	7.2
Total	1,499	455	30.4	221	14.6	784	52.4	39	2.6
Total (tables 18, 19)	15,265	4,760	31.2	2,308	15.1	7,369	48.3	828	5.4
Our material	6,658	3,111	46.7	1,147	17.1	1,993	29.9	413	6.2

Table 20. Malignant tumors

Author(s)	Age years	Total cases	Vulva	Vagina	Uterine cervix	Corpus uteri	Ovary	Tube	Breast	Gastro-intestinal tract	Other
Ahumada et al. (126)	60	88	18	–	8	18	9	1	33	–	1
Bailo et al. (135b)	60	197	14	–	25	100	40	–	14	4	–
Berger et al. (140)	60	307	79	–	25	125	46	–	–	3	32
Boguña et al. (144)	60	37	2	–	14	16	2	–	–	3	–
Camplani (151)	60	16	–	–	–	7	9	–	–	–	–
Fioretti and Andriani (171)	60	25	5	–	9	4	5	–	1	1	–
Hilfrich et al. (180)	60	117	5	–	13	73	18	–	–	–	8
Krango et al. (209)	60	38	1	–	11	14	12	–	–	–	–
Lucisano (225)	60	103	21	–	9	44	23	1	3	2	2
Mai (227)	60	62	3	–	8	21	13	–	8	–	9
Malato and Arienzo (228)	60	28	3	–	7	10	7	–	1	–	–
Mengaldo (235)	60	9	1	–	2	6	–	–	–	–	–
Noci et al. (247)	60	34	–	1	26	3	–	–	–	3	1
Polito et al. (260)	60	41	2	–	12	17	8	–	1	1	1
Rieppi et al. (266)	60	71	–	–	–	21	46	1	1	2	1
Rio (268)	60	7	–	–	1	3	1	–	2	–	–
Rusch (271)	60	223	34	–	20	73	35	–	19	–	42
Skiftis et al. (281)	60	154	26	–	–	37	91	1	–	–	–
Soferman et al. (283)	60	53	4	–	4	33	11	1	–	–	–
Stanca et al. (286)	60	32	1	–	10	17	–	2	1	1	–
Suonoja et al. (293)	60	98	–	–	15	36	47	–	–	–	–
Tancinco-Yambao and Lopez (298)	60	5	–	–	2	3	–	–	–	–	–
Trebicka (302)	60	22	1	–	2	10	8	–	–	1	–
Arenas and Bettinotti (132)	65	37	4	–	5	11	1	–	16	–	–
Bagnati and Villamayor (134)	65	21	–	–	6	11	4	–	–	–	–

Bourg and Piton (148)	65	13	2	—	2	5	—	—	4	—	—
Bulfoni et al. (150)	65	72	31	—	3	22	14	—	—	—	2
Decio (163)	65	61	7	1	16	28	7	2	—	—	—
Iwaszkiewicz (188)	65	8	—	—	—	2	6	—	—	—	—
Krupa et al. (210)	65	58	1	—	18	28	12	—	—	—	—
McKeithen (234)	65	40	—	—	—	30	8	1	—	1	—
Navratil (244)	65	194	47	1	20	53	59	1	—	—	14
Niesert and Seidenschnur (245)	65	86	16	1	10	39	16	—	—	—	4
Paldi et al. (251)	65	46	8	—	3	16	19	—	—	—	—
Piton (258)	65	31	6	1	4	13	3	—	4	—	—
Sirtori (280)	65	31	10[1]	?	4	4	12	—	1	—	1
Woraschk (319)	65	75	27	—	5	15	24	—	3	—	—
Bentzen and Anker (139)	70	20	1	—	2	10	7	—	—	—	—
Carroll and Stoddard (153)	70	18	3	—	—	5	10	—	—	—	—
Lewis (220)	70	86	28	—	4	40	10	—	—	2	2
Schilling and Schneck (274)	70	51	15	—	2	11	23	—	—	—	—
Widholm et al. (314)	70	82	22	—	—	11	44	—	—	4	1
Total	—	2,797	448	4	327	1,045	710	9	111	23	120
Our material	60	3,111	87	15	326	761	603	28	1,125	100	66

[1] Also vagina.

The differences are also partly due to the fact that many authors have only taken into account the 'large' gynecological interventions. The anesthesia in smaller gynecological operations is mentioned for example by *Horn et al.* (184) as well as *Zeman and Davids* (321). The different kinds of anesthesia in individual gynecological interventions are referred to in only a few papers (e.g. 307).

Several authors do not only list different methods of anesthesia, but also deal with the attitude of their hospital to particular anesthetic procedures (174, 176, 184, 210, 227, 255, 263, 274, 276). With regard to the details of the development of modern techniques of anesthesia, we refer to the papers mentioned here. A trend to endotracheal intubation anesthesia is unmistakable. We have not yet found any studies on the application of neuroleptic analgesia in geriatric gynecological patients.

The low proportion of anesthetic incidents in the postoperative mortality both in the literature and in our material clearly shows that the anesthetists have already been able to cope very well with geriatric operations. The cooperation of the anesthetists with the gynecologists does not end today with the end of the operation of anesthesia. We have pointed out elsewhere (199) the possibilities of joint efforts to lower further the early postoperative mortality.

Kind of Disease

In the literature, the indications for surgery are collected in various schemata. The following division appears to be most suitable: (1) malignant tumors, (2) benign tumors, (3) genital displacements, (4) other diseases.

We have collected the papers with corresponding data in tables 18 and 19. The relations are almost constant. No differences are visible, even between the age groups. The malignant tumors constitute the indication for operation in 30.4%, the benign tumors in 15.1%, the genital displacements in 49.2% and the other diseases in 5.3%.

We have found information on malignant tumors in 42 communications (table 20). At the head of the 2,797 malignancies is corpus carcinoma (1,047 cases), followed by malignant ovarian tumors (710 cases), vulvar carcinoma (448 cases) and carcinoma of the uterine cervix (327 cases). It must be taken into account here that in the two latter carcinomas radiation is often preferred at an advanced age. The different attitudes of the gynecological departments to vaginal or abdominal procedure in surgical treatment of collum carcinoma can be seen from table 21.

Our knowledge on the frequency of operation on individual tumors in various stages of life is confirmed: with increasing age, cervical carcinoma occur relatively less frequently, malignant ovarian tumors, vulvar carcinoma and corpus carcinoma, on the other hand, are a more frequent indication for surgery.

Table 21. Radical operations in collum carcinoma in geriatric operation material

Author(s)	Age years	Schauta's operation	Wertheim's operation
Arenas and Bettinotti (132)	65	0	3
Bailo et al. (135b)	60	8	30
Belopavlovič et al. (137)	60	0	13
Blanchard and Regueira (142)	60	0	7
Boguňa et al. (144)	60	0	5
Bulfoni et al. (150)	65	0	3
Decio (163)	65	6	10
Fioretti and Andriani (171)	60	3	2
Gierdal and Butters (176)	60	55	3
Hilfrich et al. (180)	60	0	2
Koláŕová and Staníček (206)	60	5	17
Loskant (224)	60	0	1
Lucisano (225)	60	0	2
Macků and Kubečka (226)	70	0	1
Mengaldo (235)	60	0	2
Navratil (244)	65	13	1
Niesert and Seidenschnur (245)	65	10	1
Polito et al. (260)	60	10	3
Randow and Riess (263)	60	24	0
Rusch (271)	60	0	20
Stanca et al. (286)	60	6	3
Szendi and Lakatos (296)	60	5	6
Vácha (306)	60	31	91
Verrelli (310)	60	0	5
Our material	60	97	108

Whereas the other malignancies of the sex organs appear sporadically, the 111 cases of mammary carcinomas are not representative (194). The gynecologist is certainly most frequently confronted with breast cancer in specific preventive examinations. A further increase in breast operations must thus be expected in gynecological operation material. The mammary carcinoma diagnosed by a gynecologist should also be operated on by him.

Ovarian tumors and uterus myomatosus constitute the overwhelming majority of benign tumors (table 22). Displacement of the uterus and vagina with or without urinary incontinence are also frequently encountered. The 'other diseases' are mostly diseases of the vulva, then various hernias, genital fistulae etc. Laparotomies because of uterine perforation have also been mentioned in some studies. A comparison of all three disease groups in a table was not possible.

Table 22. Benign tumors in geriatric gynecological operations

Author(s)	Age over years	Total cases	Benign tumors		
			cases	uterine myoma	ovarian tumors
Ahumada et al. (126)	60	165	15	1	7
Bailo et al. (135b)	60	676	90	45	43
Berger et al. (140)	60	681	134	52	82
Camplani (151)	60	157	24	4	20
Fioretti and Andriani (171)	60	144	11	3	8
Hilfrich et al. (180)	60	249	42	13	29
Kolářová and Staníček (206)	60	375	30	30	2
Krango et al. (209)	60	215	30	12	18
Lucisano (225)	60	345	45	17	25
Mai (227)	60	248	66	28	38
Malato and Arienzo (228)	60	109	39	16	7
Mengaldo (235)	60	100	11	4	7
Pernecker (255)	60	1,550	90	45	45
Polito et al. (260)	60	168	3	3	0
Rieppi et al. (266)	60	532	45	8	29
Rio (268)	60	73	9	4	5
Rusch (271)	60	1,000	70	21	43
Skiftis et al. (281)	60	398	75	20	55
Stanca et al. (286)	60	155	8	3	5
Suonoja et al. (293)	60	573	78	22	56
Trebicka (302)	60	124	23	4	19
Verrelli (310)	60	320	39	17	21
Total	60	8,357	997	372	564
Arenas and Bettinotti (132)	65	100	8	1	0
Bagnati and Villamayor (134)	65	92	12	4	8
Decio (163)	65	139	11	7	4
Iwaszkiewicz (188)	65	34	2	0	2
McKeithen (234)	65	185	25	12	13
Navratil (244)	65	474	95	26	69
Niesert and Seidenschnur (245)	65	227	24	5	19
Paldi et al. (251)	65	239	28	8	19
Piton (258)	65	110	13	6	4
Sirtori (280)	65	129	11	2	7
Tancinco-Yambao and Lopez (298)	65	99	17	3	14
Woraschk (319)	65	163	30	4	26
Total	65	1,991	276	78	185

Table 22 (continued)

Author(s)	Age over years	Total cases	Benign tumors		
			cases	uterine myoma	ovarian tumors
Bentzen and Anker (139)	70	99	5	1	4
Carroll and Stoddard (153)	70	112	3	3	0
Schilling and Schneck (174)	70	114	27	4	23
Widholm et al. (314)	70	309	71	11	56
Total	70	634	106	19	83
Total	–	10,982	1,419	469	835

Table 23. Kind of operation

Author(s)	Total cases[1]	Laparotomies		Vaginal operations and vulvar operations	
		n	%	n	%
Studies on 60-year-old female patients					
Alicino and Pietrojusti (127)	120	40	33.3	80	66.7
Bailo et al. (135b)	715	301	42.9	400	57.1
Berger et al. (140)	681	353	52.0	328	48.0
Berle et al. (141)	1,514	615	54.8	508	45.2
Blanchard and Regueira (142)	78	31	39.8	47	60.2
Boguňa et al. (144)	140	33	23.6	107	76.4
Dlhoš (165)	194	28	14.4	166	85.6
Fioretti and Andriani (171)	144	30	20.8	113	79.2
Geneja et al. (174)	299	138	46.2	161	53.8
Gierdal and Butters (176)	686	244	35.5	442	64.5
Hilfrich et al. (180)	249	150	60.2	99	39.8
Károlyi (202)	76	10	13.2	66	86.8
Kolářová and Staníček (206)	375	160	44.6	197	53.7
Krango et al. (209)	215	72	33.5	143	66.5
Lash (212)	321	77	23.9	244	76.1
Lopatecki et al. (222)	60	10	16.6	50	83.4
Loskant (224)	200	78	42.2	107	57.8
Lucisano (225)	345	123	35.9	219	64.1
Mai (227)	235	137	60.3	90	39.7
Malato and Arienzo (228)	109	50	46.0	59	54.0
Maurizio and Pescetto (231)	81	43	53.1	38	46.9

[1] Breast operations are also taken into account here.

Table 23 (continued)

Author(s)	Total cases[1]	Laparotomies		Vaginal operations and vulvar operations	
		n	%	n	%
Mengaldo (235)	100	10	10.0	90	90.0
Mirkov and Atanasov (238)	182	110	61.1	72	38.9
Pernecker (255)	1,550	429	31.0	954	69.0
Piechowiak et al. (256)	228	80	35.0	148	65.0
Polito et al. (260)	167	23	13.8	144	86.2
Randow and Riess (263)	633	325	51.6	308	48.4
Rieppi et al. (266)	532	113	21.3	419	78.7
Rio (268)	71	13	18.3	58	81.7
Rusch (271)	475	246	52.0	229	48.0
Skiftis et al. (281)	398	214	53.7	184	46.3
Stanca et al. (286)	155	22	14.3	132	85.7
Štefánik (289)	767	209	27.3	558	72.7
Suonoja et al. (293)	573	183	35.6	331	64.4
Szendi and Lakatos (296)	418	107	29.0	262	71.0
Trebicka (302)	124	49	39.8	75	60.2
Trnka (303)	564	223	39.7	341	60.3
Vácha (306)	4,313	1,536	35.6	2,777	64.1
Vácha and Stožický (307)	161	88	54.6	73	45.4
Verrelli (311)	320	100	31.2	220	68.8
Wittlinger (318)	212	101	47.9	111	52.1
Total	18,780	6,904	38.2	11,150	61.8

Studies on 65-year-old female patients

Arenas and Bettinotti (132)	76	17	22.4	59	77.6
Bagnati and Villamayor (134)	92	30	32.6	62	67.4
Bourg and Piton (148)	35	14	40.0	21	60.0
Curiel and Morresi (159)	479	44	9.2	435	90.8
Decio (163)	139	42	31.0	97	69.0
Douglas and Studdiford (167)	139	47	33.8	92	66.2
Iwaszkiewicz (188)	34	11	32.4	23	67.6
Krupa et al. (210)	181	67	37.0	114	63.0
Lefèvre (216)	111	37	33.4	74	66.6
McKeithen (234)	185	73	39.4	112	60.6
Muth (241)	213	44	20.6	169	79.4
	299	96	41.2	137	58.8
Navratil (244)	474	207	43.6	267	56.4
Niesert and Seidenschnur (245)	227	52	22.9	175	77.1

[1] Breast operations are also taken into account here.

Table 23 (continued)

Author(s)	Total cases[1]	Laparotomies		Vaginal operations and vulvar operations	
		n	%	n	%
Paldi et al. (251)	239	73	30.6	166	69.4
Piton (258)	110	41	38.7	65	61.3
Sirtori (280)	129	31	24.8	94	75.2
Tancer and Matseoane (297)	130	44	33.9	86	66.1
Tancinco-Yambao and Lopez (298)	103	33	32.0	70	68.0
Total	3,395	1,003	30.2	2,318	69.8
Studies on 70-year-old female patients					
Bentzen and Anker (139)	100	25	25.0	75	75.0
Carroll and Stoddard (153)	112	18	16.1	94	83.9
Dieminger (164)	142	64	46.8	73	53.2
Lewis (220)	316	85	26.9	231	73.1
Macků and Kubečka (226)	161	75	46.5	86	53.5
Rupprecht and Stange (270)	399	165	41.3	234	58.7
Schilling and Schneck (274)	114	55	48.2	59	51.8
Wendl (313)	129	57	48.7	60	51.3
Widholm et al. (314)	309	139	45.0	170	55.0
Total	1,782	683	38.8	1,082	61.2
Total	23,957	8,590	37.1	14,550	62.9
Our material	6,658	3,075	55.6	2,458	44.4

[1] Breast operations are also taken into account here.

Kind of Operation

The very often only global data in the literature only permitted classification of the methods of surgery in table 23 into two groups: laparotomies (37.1%) and vaginal operations with operations on the vulva (62.9%). We regard separation of the operation on the vulva from vaginal operations as expedient. However, it could not be carried out on the basis of the available literature.

We could not find any regular principle in the individual age groups. A relative increase of the laparotomies in higher age groups was found only in the paper of *Kolářová and Staníček* (206): in 60- to 69-year-old patients the vaginal

Table 24. Exploratory laparotomies in geriatric gynecological operations

Author(s)	Age years	Total cases	Laparot-omies	Exploratory laparotomies	
				n	%
Bagnati and Villamayor (134)	65	92	30	3	10.0
Bailo et al. (135b)	60	708	301	14	4.7
Belopavlovič et al. (137)	60	545	171	14	8.2
Berger et al. (140)	60	681	353	8	2.3
Blanchard and Regueira (142)	60	78	31	1	3.2
Boguña et al. (144)	60	140	33	6	18.2
Camplani (151)	60	157	46	2	4.3
Carroll and Stoddard (153)	70	112	18	8	44.4
Decio (163)	65	134	42	2	4.8
Dieminger (164)	70	142	64	19	29.7
Douglas and Studdiford (167)	65	139	47	2	4.3
Fioretti and Andriani (171)	59	144	30	4	13.3
Geneja et al. (174)	60	299	149	18	12.5
Gierdal and Butters (176)	60	686	244	27	11.1
Hilfrich et al. (180)	60	249	150	7	4.7
Károlyi (202)	60	76	10	11	10.0
Kolářová and Staníček (206)	60	375	160	18	11.3
Krupa et al. (210)	65	181	67	9	13.4
Lash (212)	60	313	77	8	10.4
Lucisano (225)	60	100	13	1	14.3
Macků and Kubečka (226)	70	161	75	16	21.3
Maurizio and Pescetto (231)	60	81	43	2	4.6
Mengaldo (235)	60	100	13	1	7.7
Muth (241)	65	299	96	12	12.5
Navratil (244)	65	474	207	24	11.6
Niesert and Seidenschnur (245)	65	227	52	8	15.4
Paldi et al. (251)	65	239	73	14	19.2
Pernecker (255)	60	1,550	429	55	12.8
Piton (258)	65	110	35	1	2.9
Randow and Riess (263)	60	633	325	22	6.8
Rieppi et al. (266)	60	532	113	9	8.0
Rigó and Zubek (267)	60	128	91	16	17.6
Rusch (271)	60	496	246	41	16.7
Schilling and Schneck (274)	70	114	51	14	27.5
Sirtori (280)	65	129	31	2	6.5
Stanca et al. (286)	60	155	22	1	4.5
Suonoja et al. (293)	60	573	183	23	12.6
Tancer and Matseoane (297)	65	130	44	3	6.8
Trebicka (302)	60	124	49	8	16.3
Trnka (303)	60	564	223	31	13.8
Uzel and Kolářová (305)	80	19	10	3	30.0
Vácha (306)	60	4,848	1,536	258	16.8

Table 24 (continued)

Author(s)	Age years	Total cases	Laparot- omies	Exploratory laparotomies	
				n	%
Verrelli (311)	60	320	100	6	6.0
Widholm et al. (314)	70	309	139	19	13.7
Wittlinger (318)	60	212	101	10	10.0
Zeman and Davids (321)	60	126	44	6	13.6
Our material	60	6,658	2,955	237	8.1

operations constituted 59.2%, the laparotomies 37.2% and the combined operations 3.6% of the interventions. In women 70–79 years old, vaginal operations were carried out in 41%, abdominal operations in 50% and combined operations in 9%. In the group over 80 years old, 40% of the patients underwent a vaginal operation and 60% an abdominal operation. The abdominal or abdominovaginal operations of descensus or prolapsus vaginae et uteri appear finally to have lost popularity (159, 176, 206, 225–227, 240, 254, 258, 266, 283, 302, 307).

Laparotomies are known to be associated with greater postoperative morbidity and mortality compared to the vaginal operations. It hence appears to be appropriate to break them down. In the communications so far only *Schilling and Schneck* (274) classified their abdominal operations: (1) total extirpation, (2) tumor extirpation, (3) exploratory laparotomy, (4) other. *Mai* (227) designated 21 of his 137 laparotomies as palliative, and *Skiftis et al.* (281) 50 of their 214. *Pernecker* (255) mentions 9 palliative laparotomies among a total of 429. The exploratory laparotomies have been mentioned in almost all papers on surgical geriatric gynecology (table 24). *Gierdal and Butters* (176) referred 20 times to an emergency laparotomy among 244 laparotomies.

Postoperative Complications

Siliquini and Petterino (279) are so far the only authors to have been concerned exclusively with the postoperative course in 60-year-old and older gynecological patients. *Berle et al.* (141), *Ceci and Casoli* (154), *Chirico and Rubin* (155) as well as *Wittig* (316) devoted great attention to this problem. In some papers only the postoperative complications which did not have a fatal course have been included, whereas in others those with a lethal outcome have also been included. Postoperative complications have been evaluated with varying intensity by the authors. Even the listing of the most frequent complica-

tions in table 25 adequately shows the diversity of the data and how com-
plicated it is to compare them. It is difficult to attain a uniform view as to what
is a complication which is worth mentioning. Despite this, some postoperative
courses deserve our special attention. In the first place we should like to name
thromboembolism. It is known that it occurs more frequently in women than in
men and that its incidence rises with increasing age. *Ardelt et al.* (131), *Wille et
al.* (315) as well as *Novotný and Dvořák* (249) have recently treated this
problem from a gynecological point of view.

Cardiovascular complications are not to be underestimated. The alterations
due to age are mostly already known here before the surgical intervention. The
best preventive for postoperative complications is hence surely thorough preoperative treatment and careful assessment of the risk of operation.

It is difficult to make a uniform interpretation of disturbed wound healing.
It is doubtful whether superficial dehiscences have already been registered
always both in vaginal operations and in laparotomies. Urogenital complications occur especially frequently in vaginal operations. Their treatment mostly
constitutes no particular problem today.

The frequency of the individual complications has altered in the course of
time. This is proved for example by the material of *Braitenberg* (149): 'Among
the complications which have occurred, the disturbed course of wound healing
and thromboses are the most important, whereas the complications such as

Table 25. Postoperative complications

Author(s)	Cases	Postoperative complications
Ahumada et al. (126)	165	infection 18, postoperative shock 4, 'organ insufficiency' 8, etc.
Alicino and Pietrojusti (127)	120	cystitis 10 (8.3%), bronchitis 7 (5.8%)
Bentzen and Anker (139)	152	pneumonia 3, myocardial infarction 2, pulmonary embolism 2, genital fistula 2, thrombophlebitis 1, visceral prolapse 1
Blanchard and Regueira (142)	87	cystitis 12 (15.3%), secondary healing 17 (21.8%), phlebitis 2 (2.6%)
Blobel and Häussler (143)	333	secondary healing 19, secondary hemorrhage 11, pulmonary embolism 4, pneumonia 2, phlebitis 1
Braitenberg (149)	325	disturbed wound healing 13 (3 visceral prolapses), thrombosis 9, circulatory failure 3, states of confusion 2, invasion of carcinoma into the intestine 2, peritonitis 2, diabetic coma 1, parotitis 1, pulmonary embolism 1

Table 25 (continued)

Author(s)	Cases	Postoperative complications
Carroll and Stoddard (153)	112	urinary retention 10, hemorrhage 2, pelveoperitonitis 2, anemia 1, perineal hematoma 1, cardiac decompensation 1, small intestinal obstruction 1, atelectasis 1, phlebitis 1
Douglas and Studdiford (167)	139	cystopyelitis 7, residual urine over 100 ml longer than 10 days after operation 6, bronchopneumonia 4, wound infection 4, senile psychosis 4, stress incontinence 3, oliguria and anuria 2, rectovaginal fistula 1, coronary thrombosis 2, wound dehiscence 2, volvulus 1, urinary bladder atonia 1, uremia 2, diabetic acidosis 1, cardiac decompensation 1, paralytic ileus 1
Horn et al. (184)	410	thromboembolism 10, phlebitis 8, disturbed wound healing 8, bronchitis 4, bronchopneumonia 3, cystitis 2, visceral prolapse 1, gastric atonia 1, exudative pleuritis 1
Kolářová and Staníček (206)	375	thromboembolic disease 5.0%, cardiovascular complications 3.0%, complications in the intestinal system 1.9%, secondary healing 1.7%, complications of the respiratory system 0.7%
Lucisano (225)	345	complications of the uropoietic tract 32, disturbed wound healing or visceral prolapse 17, pneumonia 10, cardiovascular collapse 6, allergic erythema 6, phlebitis 6, pulmonary embolism 3, shock 3, hemorrhage 3, cerebral thrombosis 2, cardiac decompensation 1, tumor cachexia 1, renal block after transfusion 1
Macků and Kubečka (226)	161	pulmonary complications 7, cardiovascular complications 5, thrombophlebitis 11, urological complications 7, secondary wound healing 6, parotitis 4
Mai (227)	235	cardiovascular weakness (or failure) 9.8%, thrombosis (thrombophlebitis) 6.9%, pulmonary embolism 6.0%, disturbed wound healing 4.3%, pneumonia 3.8%, bronchitis 2.6%, cystopyelitis 2.6%, ileus 0.4%, peritonitis 0.4%, renal failure 0.4%
Mengaldo (235)	100	cystitis 15, secondary wound healing 7, thrombophlebitis 6, phlebothrombosis 5
Muth (241)	512	complications in the wound region 19, cardiovascular diseases 15, pulmonary diseases 12, thromboses 9, pulmonary embolism and infarcts 9, subileus/ileus 8, uremia 4, liver disease 3, parotitis 3

Table 25 (continued)

Author(s)	Cases	Postoperative complications
Niesert and Seidenschnur (245)	227	potentially fatal complications: cardiovascular weakness 16, thromboembolism 10, pneumonia 6, apoplexy 3, paralytic ileus, severe intestinal atonia 4, strangulation ileus, peritonitis 1, visceral prolapse 1; not potentially fatal complications: anemia 27, cystopyelitis 19, suture dehiscence after drafting 11, wound infections 3, rectovaginal fistula 1, vesicovaginal fistula 1, jaundice 1, parametritis 1
Paldi et al. (251)	239	fever over 38 °C 26, urinary infection 12, urinary retention 7, wound seroma 7, ileus 4
Polito et al. (260)	168	cystitis 13.1%, cardiovascular decompensation 8.9%, bronchopneumonia 2.9%, diabetic dysregulation 2.3%, enteritis 1.7%, decubitus 1.7%, wound dehiscence 1.7%, thrombophlebitis 1.7%
Rieppi et al. (266)	532	cystitis 39, cystopyelitis 6, periphlebitis 7, wound dehiscence 15, bronchopneumonia 12, pulmonary embolism 2, myocardial infarction 2
Sirtori (280)	129	cystitis 13, secondary healing 6, thrombophlebitis 6, bronchopneumonia 4
Skiftis et al. (281)	398	cardiovascular failure 18, thrombosis, pulmonary embolism 14, disturbed wound healing 11, cystopyelitis 10, tracheobronchitis 8, pneumonia 4, peritonitis 1, ileus 1, parotitis 1
Štefánik (289)	367	urinary tract 12.3%, vascular system 9.3%, respiratory tract 5.7%, gastrointestinal tract 4.9%
Suonoja et al. (293)	573	fever 38 °C 94 (16.4%), poor wound healing 24 (4.2%), ileus 9 (1.6%), myocardial infarction decompensation 9 (1.6%), thromboembolism 8 (1.4%)
Tancer and Matseoane (297)	84	cystitis 4, bronchopneumonia 3, acute glaucoma 2, poor wound healing 3, cardiac complication 2, others 4
Verrelli (310)	320	cystitis 13, disturbed wound healing 11, pulmonary embolism 8, diarrhea 6, peritonitis 4, bronchopneumonia 2, thrombophlebitis 2, cardiac collapse 2, ileus 1
Wittlinger (317)	212	disturbances of wound healing 24 (11.3%), urinary tract infections 14 (6.6%), thromboembolic complications 10 (6.1%) (3 pulmonary emboli), cardiac insufficiency 7 (3.3%), pneumonia 4 (1.9%), subileus, ileus 3 (1.4%)

pneumonia and peritonitits which were formerly so feared in aged patients no longer occur.' *Vácha* (306) also observes a rapid decrease in complications of the respiratory tract, as well as good possibilities of treatment.

We list the studies with a differentiated classification of the complications in table 26. Visceral eventration is a problem with laparotomies, and intestinal complications also appear here more frequently than in vaginal operations (otherwise we could not find any appreciable differences in the two groups). Further analyses of a larger clinical material would be desirable here. *Blobel and Häussler* (143) found 9.3% postoperative complications (embolism, pneumonia, phlebitis, secondary healing, secondary bleeding) in the age group 61–65 years old, 13.4% in the group 66–70 years old, and 10% in the group 71–75 years old. Because of the small numbers, the differences are not significant. This also applies to the material of *Randow and Riess* (263). In the material of *O'Leary and Symmonds* (250), the fistulae after radical hysterectomy and pelvic eviscera-tion constitute over 50% of the complications, after radical vulvectomy and secondary healing or infiltration 71%.

The classification of the complications by *Niesert and Seidenschnur* (245) into 'potentially fatal' and 'not potentially fatal' appears worth mentioning, although even here the decision cannot always be made precisely.

In *Rigó and Zubek* (267), a 'fever state' was specified in half the postopera-tive complications. In the Mayo Clinic one speaks of a postoperative morbidity when the patients have averages of 38 °C and over at least 48 h after the first postoperative day. If this temperature persisted for only 1 postoperative day (irrespective of which), *O'Leary and Symmonds* (250) still refer to a 'non-morbid' postoperative course. This group included 90 women (67.7%) in the 133 patients operated on by them. The authors recorded a 'morbid' postoperative course in 12.1% of the radical hysterectomies, in 55% of the eventerations, and in 38.9% of the vulvectomy cases. Further data on a non-febrile and febrile postoperative course are not to be found in the geriatric gynecological literature.

Postoperative Mortality

Without exception, the postoperative mortality is analyzed or at least mentioned in all papers on surgical geriatric gynecology. It is of crucial impor-tance for the entire problem. A very high measure of comparability is especially to be aspired to here.

The time after the operation in which the death has been registered is only rarely given. The shortest time interval (10 days) was chosen by *Uhlmann* (304). *Bailo et al.* (135b) contended themselves with recording the deaths within the first 15 postoperative days. *Jäger and Pletat* (189) included all deaths which occurred within 3 weeks after his surgical intervention. After this time, only

Table 26. Postoperative complications after abdominal and vaginal interventions[1]

Author(s)	Cases	Postoperative complications
Ardelt et al. (131)	660	559 abdominal, 101 vaginal; disturbance of wound healing 12.3% (5.3%, 7%), cardiovascular disturbance 3.2% (2.1%, 1.1%), secondary bleeding 3.2% (2.1%, 1.1%), thromboembolism 2.4% (1.5%, 0.9%), visceral eventration 0.9% (0.9%), apoplectic insult 0.3% (0.3%).
Bailo et al. (135b)	708 287 (400)	pulmonary embolism and diseases of the respiratory tract 9 (14), thrombophlebitis 9 (13), cystitis 2 (19), disturbed wound healing 19 (21)
Berger et al. (140)	681	local wound complications 37 (18), cardiovascular complications 10 (2), bronchopulmonary complications 24 (15), urogenital complications 10 (12), thrombosis 10 (7), phlebitis 16 (10), peritonitis 1 (0)
Fioretti and Andriani (171)	144 27 (115)	cardiovascular collapse 0 (4), hemorrhagic shock 1 (0), pulmonary embolism 1 (1), bronchopneumonia 4 (2), thrombophlebitis 1 (4), cystitis 2 (22), disturbed wound healing 5 (26), glossitis 1 (2), acute enteritis 1 (5), decubitus 0 (3), phlebothrombosis 1 (5)
Hilfrich et al. (180)	249 150 (99)	cardiovascular decompensation 2 (3), pneumonia, bronchitis 10 (3), thrombophlebitis 5 (2), thromboembolism 9 (3), secondary healing 30 (0), visceral prolapse 4 (0), urinary tract infection 26 (18), ileus 9 (0)
Krupa et al. (210)	181	cardiovascular decompensation 2 (3), pneumonia 4 (1), phlebitis 2 (2), pulmonary embolism 1 (1), disturbed wound healing 7 (8), visceral prolapse 1 (0), urinary tract infection 2 (10)
Malato and Arienzo (228)	109 50	local complications 5 (2), bronchopulmonary complications 3 (3), decubitus 2 (1), cardiovascular complications 2 (1), vesical complications 1 (1), phlebitis 1 (1)
Piton (258)	110 45 (65)	thrombophlebitis 4 (4), disturbed wound healing 3 (5), cardiac symptoms 0 (3), respiratory complications 1 (4), diabetes 0 (2)
Randow and Riess (263)	633 325 (308)	thrombosis, thrombophlebitis 48 (26), pulmonary embolism without lethal outcome 24 (16), cardiovascular disease without lethal outcome 13 (6); pneumonia 10 (8), cystopyelitis 19 (9), peritonitis/disturbed wound healing 11 (0)
Widholm et al. (314)	309 139	wound infection 5 (0), resuture 5 (2), thrombophlebitis 3 (2), pneumonia 1 (1), myocardial infarction 1 (0), embolia in the cerebral artery 1 (0), ileus 1 (0), Douglas abscess 1 (0), pulmonary infarction 0 (1)

[1] Complications after vaginal interventions are specified in parentheses.

those cases were included which were demonstrably associated with the operation. *Cséffalvay et al.* (158), *Skiftis et al.* (281) as well as *Randow and Riess* (263) chose a period of 25 days. *Berle et al.* (141) as well as *Rupprecht and Stange* (270) registered the deaths which occurred up to the 28th postoperative day. On the other hand, *Navratil* (244), *Noci et al.* (247), *Schilling and Schneck* (274) as well as *Widholm et al.* (314) analyzed deaths in the first 30 postoperative days. It must be assumed that in most cases no fixed postoperative day, but the occurrence of exitus is the limit. We agree with *Strobel* (292), who counts in the postoperative lethality all deaths which occurred during the stay in hospital after operation, irrespective of the time lapse between operation and death. *Fioretti and Andriani* (171) have also included two deaths in which the patients died at home on the 14th day after operation.

Data on autopsy are almost never found. Information on the time of death and the age of the patient is frequently lacking. Even the diagnoses and data on the kind of operation in the operated patient who died are also not always available. Only a few authors related the individual causes of death to diagnoses and methods of operation. Often the authors preferred a rectified and non-absolute mortality after subtraction of the deaths of patients with malignancies. The immediate cause of death and not the actual postoperative complication with fatal course is often included in the statistic (visceral eventration, paralytic ileus, cardiovascular failure; visceral eventration, pulmonary embolism, cardiovascular failure; pneumonia, cardiovascular failure etc.). With two complications, the causally more important is to be chosen, e.g. visveral eventration or peritonitis. Combined analyses of causes of death and the time of death after the operation are lacking. Analysis of the causes of death in individual age groups has also rarely been undertaken (e.g. 263).

Nevertheless, the available material enables a comprehensive analysis of postoperative mortality. No cause of death was registered by *Bonanno* (145) in 108 cases, *Carroll and Stoddard* (153) in 112 cases, *Gheorghiu and Iacob* (175) in 100 cases, *Károlyi* (202) in 76 cases, *Lefèvre* (216) in 111 cases, *Mengaldo* (235) in 100 cases, *Myasischev* (243) in 48 cases, *Rigó and Zubek* (267) in 128 cases, *Stanca et al.* (286) in 158 cases, and *Verrelli* (310) in 67 cases.

Tables 27 and 28 give us an overview of the presence or absence of factors specified above in individual communications as well as on the level of the postoperative mortality in studies with varying lower age limit.

The literature data indicate only a slight age dependence of postoperative mortality. *Mikulicz-Radecki* (237) is to be mentioned in this connection. He found a total mortality of 7.3% in the women aged from 61 to 85 years who had been operated on in his hospital; this was thus three times as high as the mortality of the entire operated patient material (2.2%). The mortality of the operated patients from 11 to 60 years old was 1.4%, amounting to only 20% of the mortality of the women over 60 years old. In a further analysis, *Mikulicz-*

Table 27. Data on postoperative mortality in 60-year-old and older female patients

Author(s)	Cases total	exitus n	exitus %	Autopsy	Period of evaluation days	Time of death	Age	Diagnosis	Kind of operation	Individual causes of death known counting	by diagnosis	by kind of operation
Ahumada et al. (126)	165	12	7.2	?	–	–	–	–	–	+	–	–
Alicino and Pietrojusti (127)	120	1	0.8	?	–	–	+	+	+	+	+	+
Archilei (129)	221	4	1.8	?	–	–	–	–	+	+	–	+
Ardelt et al. (131)	660	17	2.6	?	–	–	–	–	–	+	–	–
Bailo et al. (135b)	708	13	1.8	?	15	–	–	+	+	–	–	–
Belopavlovič et al. (137)	545	10	1.8	–	–	–	–	+	+	–	–	–
Belopitov (138)	200	9	4.5	?	?	?	?	+	+	+	?	?
Berger et al. (140)	681	11	1.8	?	–	+	?	+	+	+	+	+
Berle et al. (141)	1,514	48	3.2	?	28	+	+	+	+	+	–	–
Blanchard and Regueira (142)	87	1	1.3	?	–	–	–	–	–	+	–	–
Boguňa et al. (144)	140	3	2.2	?	–	–	–	+	+	+	+	+
Camplani (151)	157	4	2.5	?	–	+	+	+	+	+	+	+
Fioretti and Andriani (171)	144	6	4.2	+	?	+	+	+	+	+	+	+
Gierdal and Butters (176)	686	44	6.4	?	–	+	+	+	+	+	–	–
Hilfrich et al. (180)	249	9	3.9	?	–	–	+	+	+	+	+	+
Horn et al. (184)	233	2	0.8	?	–	+	+	+	+	+	–	–
Kolářová and Staníček (206)	375	9	2.4	?	–	+	+	+	+	+	–	–
Krango et al. (209)	215	4	1.8	?	–	–	–	+	+	+	–	–
Lash (212)	313	14	4.5	?	–	+	+	+	+	+	+	+
Lopatecki et al. (222)	60	1	1.7	?	–	–	+	+	+	+	+	+
Loskant (224)	200	6	3.0	?	–	+	+	+	+	+	+	+
Lucisano (225)	345	14	4.0	+	–	+	+	+	+	+	+	+
Mai (227)	235	24	10.2	?	–	–	–	+	+	+	–	–

Author	n										
Malato and Arienzo (228)	109	1	0.9	?	−	+	+	+	+	+	+
Maurizio and Pescetto (231)	81	2	2.5	?	−	+	+	+	+	+	+
von Mikulicz-Radecki (237)	392	29	7.3	?	?	+	−	−	−	−	−
Mussey (242)	585	3	0.6	?	?	?	?	?	?	?	?
Nobile et al. (246)	207	2	1.0	?	−	+	+	+	+	+	+
Noci et al. (247)	34	11	32.3	?	30	+	+	+	+	+	+
Polito et al. (260)	168	1	0.6	+	−	+	+	+	+	+	+
Randow and Riess (263)	633	33	5.2	?	25	−	+	+	+	+	+
Rieppi et al. (266)	532	7	1.3	?	−	+	+	+	+	+	−
Rio (268)	73	2	2.7	?	−	+	−	−	−	−	+
Rusch (271)	496	42	8.5	?	−	?	+	+	+	+	+
Sieroszewski et al. (277)	228	8	3.5	?	?	+	+	+	+	+	+
Skiftis et al. (281)	398	21	5.3	?	25	+	+	+	+	+	+
Štefánik (289)	367	2	0.5	?	−	+	+	+	+	+	+
Suonoja et al. (293)	573	5	0.9	?	−	+	+	+	+	+	+
Szendi and Lakatos (296)	418	2	0.5	?	−	?	?	?	?	?	?
Te Linde (299)	112	3	2.7	?	?	?	−	−	−	?	?
Trebicka (302)	124	2	1.6	?	−	−	−	−	−	+	+
Trnka (303)	564	14	2.3	?	−	−	−	−	+	−	−
Vácha (306)	5,348	82	1.5	?	−	+	−	+	+	−	−
Vácha and Stožický (307)	161	6	3.7	(+)	−	+	+	+	+	+	+
Verrelli (311)	253	4	1.6	−	−	+	+	+	+	+	+
Wittig (316)	528	25	4.7	−	−	(+)	(+)	+	−	−	−
Wittlinger (317)	212	5	2.4	?	−	−	−	−	−	−	−

+ = Remarks existent; − = remarks not existent; ? = no comment.

Table 28. Data on postoperative mortality in 65- and 70-year-old and older female patients

Author(s)	Cases total	exitus n	%	Autopsy	Period of evaluation days	Time of death	Age	Diagnosis	Kind of operation	Individual causes of death known counting	by diagnosis	by kind of operation
Arenas and Bettinotti (132)	100	1	1.0	?	–	–	+	+	–	+	+	–
Blanchard and Regueira (142)	78	1	1.3	?	–	+	–	–	–	+	–	–
Bourg and Piton (148)	40	5	12.5	?	?	?	–	+	+	–	–	+
Curiel and Morresi (159)	481	8	1.7	?	–	+	–	+	+	+	+	+
Decio (163)	139	2	1.4	?	–	+	+	+	+	+	+	+
Douglas (166)	163	4	3.5	?	–	+	–	–	+	+	+	–
Douglas and Studdiford (167)	139	9	6.5	+	–	–	–	+	+	+	+	+
Gause (173)	374	2	0.6	?	–	+	–	–	+	+	+	–
Iwaszkiewicz (188)	34	1	2.9	?	–	–	+	+	–	+	+	+
Krupa et al. (210)	181	4	2.2	?	–	–	–	–	–	+	–	–
Levy and Melchior (219)	476	21	4.4	?	–	–	–	–	+	–	–	–
McKeithen (234)	158	2	1.3	?	–	–	–	–	+	+	–	+
Muth (241)	213	12	5.6	?	–	–	+	+	+	+	+	+
Navratil (244)	474	38	8.0	?	30	–	–	+	+	+	+	+
Niesert and Seidenschnur (245)	227	25	11.0	?	–	–	–	+	+	+	+	+
O'Leary and Symmonds (250)	133	5	3.8	?	–	+	–	–	+	+	+	–
Paldi et al. (251)	136	1	0.7	?	–	–	+	+	+	+	+	+
Paldi et al. (252)	239	3	1.3	?	–	–	+	+	+	+	+	+
Piton (258)	110	7	6.4	+	–	–	+	+	+	+	+	+
Sirtori (280)	129	6	4.7	?	–	–	–	–	–	+	–	–
Tancer and Matseoane (297)	130	3	2.3	+	–	+	+	+	+	+	+	+
Woraschk (319)	163	12	7.8	?	–	–	–	–	–	+	–	–
Bentzen and Anker (139)	100	3	3.0	+	–	+	+	+	+	+	+	+

Reference												
Braitenberg (149)	325	11	3.4	?	−	+	+	+	+	+	−	−
Dieminger (164)	142	11	7.6	?	−	−	−	+	+	+	−	−
Lewis (220)	305	6	1.9	?	−	−	−	+	−	−	−	+
Mackú and Kubečka (226)	161	7	4.3	?	−	−	−	+	−	−	−	−
Rupprecht and Stange (270)	399	31	7.8	?	28	−	−	+	−	−	−	−
Schilling and Schneck (274)	114	7	6.1	?	30	−	+	+	−	+	−	−
Schürmann (276)	214	24	11.2	?	−	−	−	+	−	−	−	−
Uhlmann (304)	73	5	6.9	?	10	+	+	+	+	+	+	+
Uzel and Kolářová (305)[1]	19	1	5.2	?	−	+	+	+	+	+	−	+
Wendl (313)	129	7	5.5	?	−	−	+	+	−	+	+	+
Widholm et al. (314)	309	9	2.9	?	30	+	+	+	+	+	+	−

+ = Remarks existent; − = remarks not existent; ? = no comment.
[1] 80-year-old and older female patients.

Radecki (237) arrived at the view that the high mortality of the women over 60 years is 'neither due to the operation nor to age, but to fate'. The qualitatively unfavorable composition of the geriatric patient material does not justify therapeutic passivity.

In table 29, the deaths are classified according to individual disease groups. The malignant tumors constitute 64.9%, the benign tumors 10.7%, the genital displacements 14.8% and the group of 'other or unknown diseases' 9.6% of the deaths. It would be more correct to take into account the mortality proportions of all cases of the individual disease groups and not the proportion among all the postoperative deaths. In table 30, the laparotomies represent 260 deaths (69.8%), the vulva/vagina operations 99 deaths (26.9%), and other diseases 12 deaths (3.3%). The laparotomies are always numerically less than the vaginal operations. Their proportion in the total postoperative mortality is thus even higher. Unfortunately, we did not find an analysis of the deaths with different laparotomies in any communication.

Table 31 with the analysis of the causes of 458 deaths is clinically important. The number of 'anesthesia deaths' and postoperative shocks is remarkably low. Pulmonary embolism is the most frequent cause of death (178 cases, 27.5%). It is to be assumed that this diagnosis was mostly verified by autopsy. The possibilities of a successful control of fatal pulmonary embolism in elderly gynecological patients were described by *Wittig* (316) and *Ardelt et al.* (131).

With 177 cases (27.3%), 'cardiovascular failure' takes second place. The differing interpretation of this term as cause of postoperative death is interesting: *Schilling and Schneck* (274) reported that cardiovascular deaths all involve deterioration of cardiovascular diseases which were already manifest preoperatively due to the operation. *Velikay* (309) comments in the analysis of the operation material of his hospital that almost all cases which died of cardiovascular failure (51.3% of the entire mortality) had been designated as generally operable by the internist who was consulted. *Irmscher* (187) also has a similar attitude to the postoperative deaths due to 'cardiovascular failure'. As further causes of death follow tumor cachexia (72 cases), peritonitis (65 cases) and ileus (41 cases). The frequency of other fatal postoperative complications is to be seen from table 31.

In the malignant tumors (table 32), cardiovascular failure constitutes the 'predominant' cause of death with 49 cases (29.7%). This is surely associated more frequently with the terminal stage of the basic condition than with a fatal decompensation of the cardiovascular system. Peritonitis and pulmonary embolism take second and third place with 25 and 26 cases respectively, and ileus is fourth with 21 cases. The higher percentage of 'tumor cachexia' might be interpreted as a sign for the relatively late surgical intervention. The 18 cases (10.9%) are not sufficient for such an evaluation.

In the 57 recorded cases of benign tumors, pulmonary embolism was specified as the cause of death 15 times and cardiovascular failure 12 times (table 33). Very probably, autopsy was carried out more frequently in these grave fatalities, so that the 'stopgap diagnosis' cardiovascular failure was used very much more rarely. Pulmonary embolism was also at the forefront 20 times among the 48 deaths of patients operated on for genital displacement. The same explanation surely applies for the 6 cases of 'cardiovascular failure' as with the benign tumors. The 6 fatal bronchopneumonias are noteworthy.

In table 34 the following causes of death are at the forefront in laparotomies: 32 cardiovascular failures, 30 peritonitis and 28 pulmonary embolism. In the genital displacements, pulmonary embolism is in the lead with 27 cases, followed by 13 cases cardiovascular failure. 8 cases of an organic disease of the cardiovascular system are noteworthy here.

General Papers on Surgical Geriatric Gynecology Which Were Not Taken into Account

There are many papers which are concerned with problems of surgical geriatric gynecology in only general terms without evaluation of the author's own material worth mentioning (136a, 169, 181, 208, 213, 214, 230, 239, 273), while some other papers were not available to us (133, 156, 157, 170, 172, 203, 229, 261, 269, 272).

Conclusions

Division into early and late postmenopause is generally recognized. In addition to the previous views, the late postmenopause can be taken to mean the beginning of the hypohormonal phase and the senium to mean the advanced stage of the hypohormonal phase. The geriatric gynecological problems begin at the age of 60 or 65. The first phase of geriatric gynecology roughly corresponds to the late postmenopause and the second phase to the senium. Gynecological pathology is also in the forefront in older women. The designation 'geriatric gynecology' is more appropriate than 'gynecological geriatrics'. Gerontology is concerned with the physiological processes of aging. In surgical problems, one must thus speak of a 'surgical geriatric gynecology' and not of 'surgical gerontological gynecology'.

In order to make it easier to systematize the previous literature, we presented a draft of the conception 'gynecology of elderly and very old women'. It would be appropriate to separate the physiological processes of aging from diseases of the female sex organs. This requirement is met with the terms 'gerontological gynecology' and 'geriatric gynecology'.

Table 29. Fatalities and kind of diseases

Author(s)	Age years	Total cases	Fatalities		malignant tumors	benign tumors	genital displacements	unknown or other diseases
			n	%				
Belopavlovič et al. (137)	60	545	10	1.8	8	1	1	0
Berger et al. (140)	60	681	11	1.8	7	1	3	0
Fioretti and Andriani (171)	60	144	6	4.2	2	0	4	0
Gierdal and Butters (176)	60	686	44	6.4	40	?	?	4
Hilfrich et al. (180)	60	249	9	3.9	6	3	0	0
Kolářová and Staníček (206)	60	375	9	2.4	5	3	1	0
Lash (212)	60	313	14	4.5	5	2	7	9
Loskant (224)	60	200	6	3.0	5	0	0	1
Lucisano (225)	60	345	14	4.0	8	4	2	0
Mai (227)	60	235	24	10.2	10	?	?	14
Malato and Arienzo (228)	60	109	1	0.9	1	0	0	0
Maurizio and Pescetto (231)	60	81	2	2.5	1	0	1	0
von Mikulicz-Radecki (237)	61	392	29	7.3	24	2	3	–
Polito et al. (260)	60	168	1	6.0	–	–	–	1
Randow and Riess (263)	60	633	33	5.2	22	3	3	5
Rieppi et al. (266)	60	532	7	1.3	2	0	5	0
Rio (268)	60	73	2	2.7	0	1	1	0
Siliquini and Petterino (279)	60	479	4	0.8	4	0	0	0
Štefánik (289)	60	367	2	0.5	1	1	0	0
Suonoja et al. (293)	60	573	5	0.8	3	0	1	1
Szendi and Lakatos (296)	60	418	2	0.5	2	0	0	0
Trebicka (302)	60	124	2	1.6	1	1	0	0
Verrelli (311)	60	253	4	1.6	2	0	2	0
Wittlinger (317)	60	212	5	4.4	4	0	0	1
Total	60	8,187	246	3.0	163	22	34	27

Curiel and Morresi (159)	65	481	8	1.7	0	2	6	0
Decio (163)	65	139	2	1.4	2	0	0	0
Douglas and Studdiford (167)	65	139	9	6.5	6	0	3	0
Iwaszkiewicz (188)	65	34	1	2.9	1	0	0	0
Navratil (244)	65	474	38	8.0	30	6	2	0
Niesert and Seidenschnur (245)	65	227	25	11.0	13	5	6	1
Paldi et al. (251)	65	239	3	1.3	3	0	0	0
Piton (258)	65	110	7	6.4	5	0	2	0
Tancer and Matseoane (297)	65	130	3	2.3	1	1	0	1
Total	65	1,973	96	4.9	61	14	19	2
Bentzen and Anker (139)	70	100	3	3	2	0	1	0
Braitenberg (149)	70	325	11	3.4	10	0	0	1
Dieminger (164)	70	142	11	7.6	6	?	?	5
Schilling and Schneck (274)	70	114	7	6.1	5	0	2	0
Wendl (313)	70	129	7	5.5	5	?	?	2
Widholm et al. (314)	70	309	9	2.9	2	5	1	1
Total	70	1,119	48	4.3	30	5	4	9
Total	–	11,279	390	3.5	254	41	57	38
Our material	60	6,658	511	7.7	378	57	40	36

Table 30. Fatalities and kind of operation

Author(s)	Age years	Total cases	Fatalities		laparot-omies	vulva-vagina operations	unknown or other kind of operations
			n	%			
Archilei (129)	60	221	4	1.8	4	0	0
Berger et al. (140)	60	681	11	1.8	4	7	0
Berle et al. (141)	60	1,514	48	3.1	36	10	2
Fioretti and Andriani (171)	60	144	6	4.2	2	4	0
Hilfrich et al. (180)	60	249	9	3.9	9	0	0
Kolářová and Staníček (206)	60	375	9	2.4	8	1	0
Lash (212)	60	313	14	4.5	6	8	0
Loskant (224)	60	200	6	3.0	5	?	1
Lucisano (225)	60	345	14	4.0	10	4	0
Mai (227)	60	235	24	10.2	20	4	0
Malato and Arienzo (228)	60	109	1	0.9	1	0	0
Maurizio and Pescetto (231)	60	81	2	2.5	1	1	0
Polito et al. (260)	60	168	1	0.6	0	0	1
Randow and Riess (263)	60	633	33	5.2	25	8	0
Rieppi et al. (266)	60	532	7	1.3	2	5	0
Rio (268)	60	73	2	2.7	1	1	0
Štefánik (289)	60	367	2	0.5	2	1	0
Suonoja et al. (293)	60	573	5	0.8	4	0	1
Trebicka (302)	60	124	2	1.6	2	0	0
Verrelli (311)	60	253	4	1.6	3	1	0
Wittlinger (317)	60	212	5	2.4	4	1	0
Total	60	7,402	209	2.8	149	56	4

Bourg and Piton (148)	65	40	5	12.5	4	1	0
Curiel and Morresi (159)	65	481	8	1.7	2	6	0
Decio (163)	65	139	2	1.4	2	0	0
Douglas and Studdiford (167)	65	139	9	6.5	5	4	0
Iwaszkiewicz (188)	65	34	1	2.9	1	0	0
Muth (241)	65	213	12	5.6	5	7	0
Navratil (244)	65	474	38	8.0	31	7	0
Niesert and Seidenschnur (245)	65	227	25	11.0	19	6	0
O'Leary and Symmonds (250)	65	133	5	3.8	4	1	0
Paldi et al. (252)	65	239	3	1.3	3	0	0
Piton (258)	65	110	7	6.4	6	1	0
Sirtori (280)	65	101	3	3.0	1	2	0
Total	65	2,330	118	5.1	83	35	0
Bentzen and Anker (139)	70	100	3	3	1	2	0
Braitenberg (149)	70	325	11	3.4	2	1	8
Dieminger (164)	70	141	11	7.6	8	3	0
Widholm et al. (314)	70	309	9	2.9	8	1	0
Total	70	875	34	3.9	19	7	8
Total	—	10,607	361	3.4	251	98	12
Our material	60	6,658	511	7.7	426	57	28

Table 31. Individual causes of death

Author(s)	Age years	Total cases	Fatalities n	Fatalities %	Anesthetic incident and postoperative shock	Pulmonary embolism	Cardiovascular failure	Organic diseases of cardiovascular system	Bronchopneumonia	Uremia	Peritonitis, sepsis, visceral eventration	Ileus	Tumor cachexia	Other
Ahumada et al. (126)	60	165	12	7.2	3	1	2	–	–	1	1	–	1	3
Alicino and Pietrojusti (127)	60	120	1	0.8	–	1	1	–	–	–	–	–	–	–
Archilei (129)	60	221	4	1.8	–	2	1	–	1	–	–	–	–	3
Ardelt et al. (131)	60	660	17	2.6	–	2	10	–	–	1	2	–	–	1
Belopitov (138)	60	200	9	4.5	1	2	1	–	–	1	4	–	–	1
Berger et al. (140)	60	681	11	1.8	1	2	4	–	–	1	1	–	–	1
Boguña et al. (144)	60	140	3	2.2	1	–	–	2	–	–	–	–	–	–
Fioretti and Andriani (171)	60	144	6	4.2	1	–	4	–	1	–	–	–	–	–
Hilfrich et al. (180)	60	249	9	3.9	–	2	3	–	1	–	2	1	–	–
Kolářová and Staníček (206)	60	375	9	2.4	1	3	1	–	–	–	1	–	3	–
Krango et al. (209)	60	215	4	1.8	2	2	1	–	–	1	–	–	–	–
Lash (212)	60	313	14	4.5	–	1	1	–	3	1	5	–	1	–
Lopatecki et al. (222)	60	60	1	1.7	–	1	–	–	–	1	–	–	–	–
Loskant (224)	60	200	6	3.0	–	2	1	1	–	–	1	–	2	–
Lucisano (225)	60	345	14	4.1	–	3	6	3	2	–	1	–	1	–
Mai (227)	60	235	24	10.2	–	12	7	–	2	–	–	–	–	–
Malato and Arienzo (228)	60	109	1	0.9	–	1	1	–	–	–	–	–	–	–
Maurizio and Pescetto (231)	60	81	2	2.5	–	–	1	–	2	–	–	1	–	–
von Mikulicz-Radecki (237)	60	392	29	7.3	–	7	13	1	2	1	–	3	2	–
Polito et al. (260)	60	168	1	0.6	–	1	–	–	–	–	–	–	–	–

Randow and Riess (263)	60	633	33	5.2	—	16	5	—	1	4	3	1	3	—
Rieppi et al. (266)	60	532	7	1.3	—	4	2	1	—	—	—	—	—	—
Rio (268)	60	73	2	2.7	—	1	1	2	—	—	12	—	4	4
Rusch (271)	60	496	42	8.5	—	14	3	—	2	—	—	1	5	—
Sieroszewski et al. (277)	60	228	8	3.5	—	1	2	—	—	—	1	1	—	—
Skiftis et al. (281)	60	398	21	5.3	—	5	12	—	2	—	—	1	—	—
Štefánik (289)	60	367	2	0.5	1	1	—	—	—	—	1	—	1	—
Suonoja et al. (293)	60	573	5	0.8	1	1	—	1	—	—	1	1	1	—
Szendi and Lakatos (296)	60	418	2	0.5	—	—	—	1	—	—	1	—	1	—
Trebicka (302)	60	124	2	1.6	—	4	—	1	—	—	1	—	4	—
Trnka (303)	60	569	14	2.3	1	4	—	4	—	—	5	2	18	4
Vácha (306)	60	5,348	82	1.5	5	24	19	2	3	—	—	—	3	—
Vácha and Stožický (307)	60	161	6	3.7	—	2	1	—	—	—	—	1	—	—
Verrelli (311)	60	253	4	1.6	—	3	—	2	—	—	—	—	—	1
Wittlinger (317)	60	212	5	2.4	—	2	2	—	—	—	—	—	—	—
Total	60	15,458	412	2.7	17	124	103	18	18	10	43	12	49	18

Table 31. (continued)

Author(s)	Age years	Total cases	Fatalities n	Fatalities %	Anesthetic incident and postoperative shock	Pulmonary embolism	Cardiovascular failure	Organic diseases of cardiovascular system	Bronchopneumonia	Uremia	Peritonitis, sepsis, visceral eventration	Ileus	Tumor cachexia	Other
Arenas and Bettinotti (132)	65	100	1	1.0	–	–	–	–	–	1	–	–	–	–
Blanchard and Regueira (142)	65	78	1	1.3	1	–	–	–	–	–	–	–	–	–
Curiel and Morresi (159)	65	481	8	1.7	–	2	2	–	1	–	3	–	–	–
Decio (163)	65	139	2	1.4	–	1	–	–	–	–	1	–	–	–
Douglas and Studdiford (167)	65	139	9	6.5	1	–	1	3	–	–	–	2	–	2
Iwaszkiewicz (188)	65	34	1	2.9	–	–	–	–	1	–	–	–	–	–
Krupa et al. (210)	65	181	4	2.2	–	2	–	–	1	–	–	–	1	–
McKeithen (234)	65	185	2	1.1	–	1	–	–	–	–	–	–	1	–
Muth (241)	65	213	12	5.6	–	1	3	2	1	–	–	4	–	1
	65	299	10	3.3	–	–	–	–	2	–	1	5	–	2
Navratil (244)	65	474	38	8.0	–	9	8	–	3	–	8	4	6	–
Niesert and Seidenschnur (245)	65	227	25	11.0	–	5	12	–	3	–	–	1	4	–
O'Leary and Symmonds (250)	65	133	5	3.8	–	–	–	1	–	–	3	–	–	1
Paldi et al. (252)	65	239	3	1.3	–	–	–	1	–	–	–	2	–	–
Piton (258)	65	110	7	6.4	3	1	2	–	–	–	2	–	–	–
Sirtori (280)	65	101	3	3.0	–	1	1	–	–	1	–	–	–	–
Tancer and Matseoane (297)	65	130	3	2.3	–	1	1	1	–	–	–	–	–	–
Total	65	3,263	134	4.1	5	23	30	8	12	2	18	18	12	6

Reference	Year	n		%										
Bentzen and Anker (139)	70	100	3	3.0	—	—	—	1	1	1	—	—	—	—
Braitenberg (149)	70	325	11	3.4	—	5	1	—	—	—	2	—	2	1
Dieminger (164)	70	142	11	7.7	—	5	—	2	—	—	—	—	3	1
Lewis (220)	70	305	6	1.9	1	3	—	1	—	—	—	1	—	—
Mackú and Kubečka (226)	71	161	7	4.3	—	3	3	—	—	—	—	1	—	—
Rupprecht and Stange (270)	70	399	31	7.8	—	6	18	—	2	—	2	2	1	—
Schilling and Schneck (274)	70	114	7	6.1	—	2	4	—	1	—	—	—	—	—
Schürmann (276)	70	214	24	11.2	—	4	14	—	1	—	—	—	5	—
Uhlmann (304)	70	73	5	6.9	—	3	1	—	—	—	—	1	—	—
Wendl (313)	70	129	7	9.5	—	—	2	—	—	—	—	5	—	—
Widholm et al. (314)	70	309	9	2.9	—	—	1	—	4	—	3	1	—	—
Total	70	2,271	121	5.3	1	31	44	4	9	1	7	11	11	2
Total	—	20,992	667	3.2	23	178	177	30	39	13	68	41	72	26
Our material	60	6,658	511	7.7	25	90	103	35	44	18	72	35	75	14

Table 32. Causes of death in malignant tumors

Author(s)	Age years	Total cases	Fatalities n	Fatalities %	Anesthetic incident and postoperative shock	Pulmonary embolism	Cardiovascular failure	Organic diseases of cardiovascular system	Bronchopneumonia	Uremia	Peritonitis, sepsis, visceral eventration	Ileus	Tumor cachexia	Other
Alicino and Pietrojusti (127)	60	?	1	?	—	—	1	—	—	—	—	—	—	—
Bentzen and Anker (139)	70	20	2	10.0	—	—	—	—	1	—	1	—	—	—
Berger et al. (140)	60	307	7	2.3	1	1	4	1	—	—	—	—	—	—
Braitenberg (149)	70	?	10	?	—	5	1	—	—	—	1	—	2	1
Decio (163)	65	61	2	3.3	—	1	1	1	—	—	1	—	—	—
Douglas and Studdiford (167)	65	?	6	?	1	—	1	—	—	—	—	2	—	1
Fioretti and Andriani (171)	60	25	2	8.0	1	—	1	—	—	—	—	—	—	—
Hilfrich et al. (180)	60	117	6	5.1	—	—	3	—	—	—	2	1	—	—
Iwaszkiewicz (188)	65	8	1	12.5	—	—	1	—	—	—	—	—	1	—
Kolářová and Staníček (206)	60	170	5	3.0	1	—	—	—	—	—	—	—	3	—
Lash (212)	60	?	5	?	1	—	1	—	—	—	3	—	1	—
Loskant (224)	60	?	5	?	—	2	—	—	—	—	1	—	2	—
Lucisano (225)	60	103	8	7.7	—	—	5	1	—	—	1	—	1	—
Malato and Arienzo (228)	60	28	1	3.6	—	1	—	—	—	—	—	—	—	—
Maurizio and Pescetto (231)	60	?	1	?	—	—	1	—	—	—	—	—	—	—
von Mikulicz-Radecki (237)	61	?	24	?	—	3	13	1	1	1	—	3	2	—
Navratil (244)	65	194	30	15.5	—	5	7	1	2	—	7	5	4	—
Noci et al. (247)	60	34	11	3.2	—	3	3	2	—	1	2	—	—	—
O'Leary and Symmonds (250)	65	133	5	3.8	—	1	—	1	—	—	3	—	—	1
Paldi et al. (251)	65	46	3	6.6	—	—	—	—	—	—	—	2	—	—

	A	B	C	D	E	F	G	H	I	J	K	L	M	N
Piton (258)	65	31	5	15.8	3	—	1	—	—	—	—	1	—	—
Rieppi et al. (266)	60	71	2	2.8	—	1	2	—	—	—	—	—	—	—
Schilling and Schneck (274)	70	51	5	9.8	—	1	3	—	—	—	1	—	—	—
Štefánik (289)	60	70	1	1.4	1	—	—	—	—	—	1	—	1	—
Suonoja et al. (293)	60	98	3	3.1	1	—	—	—	—	—	1	1	1	—
Szendi and Lakatos (296)	60	132	2	1.5	—	—	1	—	—	—	1	1	1	—
Tancer and Matseoane (297)	65	?	1	?	—	—	—	—	—	—	—	—	1	—
Trebicka (302)	60	22	1	4.5	—	—	—	—	—	—	—	—	—	—
Verrelli (311)	60	?	2	?	—	2	—	—	—	—	—	—	—	—
Wendl (313)	70	?	5	?	—	—	—	—	—	—	—	5	—	—
Widholm et al. (314)	70	82	2	2.4	—	—	—	—	1	—	1	—	—	—
Total	—	—	164	—	10	25	48	7	5	2	26	20	18	3
Our material	60	3,111	377	12.1	18	52	82	22	37	11	49	22	75	9

Table 33. Causes of death in benign tumors, genital displacements and other as well as unknown diseases

Author(s)	Age years	Total cases	Fatalities n	Fatalities %	Anesthetic incident and postoperative shock	Pulmonary embolism	Cardiovascular failure	Organic diseases of cardiovascular system	Bronchopneumonia	Uremia	Peritonitis, sepsis, visceral eventration	Ileus	Other
Benign tumors													
Berger et al. (140)	60	138	1	0.7	–	–	–	–	–	–	1	–	–
Curiel and Morresi (159)	65	92	2	2.2	–	–	1	–	–	–	1	–	–
Hilfrich et al. (180)	60	42	3	7.1	–	2	–	–	1	–	–	–	–
Kolářová and Staníček (206)	60	30	2	6.7	–	2	–	–	–	–	–	–	–
Lash (212)	60	?	2	?	1	–	–	–	–	–	1	–	–
Lucisano (225)	60	45	4	8.9	–	1	1	2	–	–	–	–	–
von Mikulicz-Radecki (237)	61	?	2	?	–	1	–	–	1	–	–	–	–
Navratil (244)	65	95	6	6.3	–	2	1	–	1	–	1	1	–
Randow and Riess (263)	60	?	3	?	–	3	–	–	–	–	–	–	–
Rio (268)	60	9	1	11.1	–	1	–	–	–	–	–	–	–
Štefánik (289)	60	44	1	2.3	–	1	–	–	–	–	–	–	–
Tancer and Matseoane (297)	65	?	1	?	–	–	–	1	–	–	–	–	–
Trebicka (302)	60	23	1	4.4	–	1	–	–	–	–	–	–	–
Widholm et al. (314)	70	71	5	7.0	–	–	1	–	1	1	1	1	–
Total	–	–	34	–	1	14	4	3	4	1	5	2	–
Our material	60	1,141	57	4.7	5	15	12	4	1	2	7	9	2

Genital displacements

Reference		n	%									
Bentzen and Anker (139)	70	5	2.0	—	—	—	—	—	—	—	—	—
Berger et al. (140)	60	236	1.3	—	1	—	1	1	—	—	—	1
Curiel and Morresi (159)	65	388	1.5	—	2	1	1	2	—	2	—	1
Douglas and Studdiford (167)	65	?	?	—	—	—	2	—	—	—	—	—
Fioretti and Andriani (171)	60	95	4.2	—	1	3	1	—	—	—	—	—
Kolářová and Staníček (206)	60	135	0.7	—	1	—	—	1	—	1	—	—
Lash (212)	60	?	?	1	1	—	—	1	1	—	—	—
Lucisano (225)	60	167	1.2	—	2	—	—	—	—	—	—	—
Maurizio and Pescetto (231)	60	38	2.6	—	1	—	—	—	—	—	—	—
von Mikulicz-Radecki (237)	61	?	?	—	3	—	—	—	—	—	—	—
Navratil (244)	65	162	1.2	1	2	—	—	—	—	—	—	—
Piton (258)	65	53	3.8	—	—	—	1	—	—	—	1	—
Rieppi et al. (266)	60	412	1.2	—	4	—	1	1	1	—	—	—
Rio (268)	60	45	2.2	—	—	—	—	—	—	—	—	—
Schilling and Schneck (274)	70	34	5.9	—	1	1	1	—	—	—	—	—
Suonoja et al. (293)	60	367	0.3	—	1	1	—	—	—	—	—	—
Verrelli (311)	60	?	?	—	1	—	—	—	—	1	1	—
Widholm et al. (314)	70	134	0.7	—	—	—	—	—	—	—	—	—
Wittlinger (318)	60	114	0.9	—	—	—	—	—	—	—	—	1
Total	—	—	48	2	20	6	5	6	1	3	2	3
Our material	60	1,993	2.0	1	18	3	8	4	2	3	2	2

Table 33 (continued)

Author(s)	Age years	Total cases	Fatalities n	Fatalities %	Anesthetic incident and postoperative shock	Pulmonary embolism	Cardiovascular failure	Organic diseases of cardiovascular system	Bronchopneumonia	Uremia	Peritonitis, sepsis, visceral eventration	Ileus	Other
Other diseases													
Braitenberg (149)	70	?	1	?	–	–	–	–	–	–	1	–	–
Kolářová and Staníček (206)	60	40	1	2.5	–	–	–	–	–	–	1	–	–
Loskant (224)	60	?	1	?	–	–	–	1	–	–	–	–	–
Polito et al. (260)	60	168	1	0.6	–	1	–	–	–	–	–	–	–
Suonoja et al. (293)	60	30	1	3.3	–	–	–	1	–	–	–	–	–
Tancer and Matseoane (297)	65	?	1	?	–	–	–	1	–	–	–	–	–
Widholm et al. (314)	70	22	1	4.5	–	–	–	–	1	–	–	–	–
Total	–	–	7	–	–	1	–	3	1	–	2	–	–
Our material	60	413	37	9.0	1	5	6	1	2	3	14	4	1

Table 34. Causes of death in laparotomies, vulva and vagina operations as well as in unknown kinds of operations

Author(s)	Age years	Total cases	Fatalities n	Fatalities %	Anesthetic incident and postoperative shock	Pulmonary embolism	Cardiovascular failure	Organic diseases of cardiovascular system	Bronchopneumonia	Uremia	Peritonitis, sepsis, visceral eventration	Ileus	Tumor cachexia	Other
Laparotomies														
Alicino and Pietrojusti (127)	60	40	1	2.5	–	–	1	–	–	–	–	–	–	–
Archilei (129)	60	46	4	8.7	–	2	1	–	1	–	–	–	–	–
Bentzen and Anker (139)	70	25	1	4.0	–	–	–	1	–	–	–	–	–	–
Berger et al. (140)	60	353	4	1.1	–	–	2	–	–	–	2	–	–	–
Braitenberg (149)	70	?	2	?	–	–	1	–	–	–	1	–	–	–
Curiel and Morresi (159)	65	44	2	4.5	–	1	1	–	–	–	–	–	–	–
Decio (163)	65	42	2	4.8	–	–	–	–	–	–	2	–	–	–
Douglas and Studdiford (167)	65	47	5	10.7	1	–	1	–	–	–	2	–	–	1
Fioretti and Andriani (171)	60	30	2	6.7	1	–	–	–	1	–	–	–	–	–
Hilfrich et al. (180)	60	150	9	6.0	–	2	3	–	1	–	2	1	–	–
Iwaszkiewicz (188)	65	11	1	9.0	–	–	–	–	–	–	–	–	1	–
Kolářová and Staníček (206)	60	160	8	5.0	1	2	1	–	–	–	1	–	3	–
Lash (212)	60	77	6	7.8	1	–	1	–	–	–	3	–	1	–
Loskant (224)	60	78	4	5.1	–	1	–	–	–	–	1	–	2	–
Lucisano (225)	60	123	10	8.1	–	–	6	2	–	–	1	–	1	–
Malato and Arienzo (228)	60	50	1	2.0	–	1	–	–	–	–	–	–	–	–
Maurizio and Pescetto (231)	60	43	1	2.3	–	–	1	–	–	–	–	–	–	–
Navratil (244)	65	207	31	15.0	–	4	7	–	3	–	8	6	3	–

Table 34 (continued)

Author(s)	Age years	Total cases	Fatalities n	Fatalities %	Anesthetic incident and postoperative shock	Pulmonary embolism	Cardiovascular failure	Organic diseases of cardiovascular system	Bronchopneumonia	Uremia	Peritonitis, sepsis, visceral eventration	Ileus	Tumor cachexia	Other
O'Leary and Symmonds (250)	65	61	4	6.6	–	–	–	–	–	–	3	–	–	1
Paldi et al. (251)	65	73	3	4.1	–	–	–	1	–	–	–	2	–	–
Piton (258)	65	41	6	15.0	3	–	1	–	–	–	–	2	–	–
Randow and Riess (263)	60	325	25	7.7	–	10	3	–	1	4	3	1	3	–
Rieppi et al. (266)	60	113	2	1.8	–	–	2	–	–	–	–	–	–	–
Rio (268)	60	12	1	8.3	–	1	–	–	–	–	–	–	–	–
Štefánik (289)	60	209	2	1.0	1	–	–	1	–	–	–	–	–	–
Suonoja et al. (293)	60	183	4	2.2	1	–	–	1	–	–	1	–	1	–
Szendi and Lakatos (296)	60	107	1	0.9	–	–	–	1	–	–	–	–	–	–
Tancer and Matseoane (297)	65	44	3	6.8	–	1	1	1	–	–	–	–	–	–
Trebicka (302)	60	49	2	4.0	–	–	–	–	–	–	–	1	1	–
Verrelli (311)	60	100	3	3.0	–	2	–	–	–	–	–	1	–	–
Total	–	–	150	–	9	28	32	7	7	4	31	14	16	2
Our material	60	3,269	431	13.2	22	63	92	15	37	16	67	34	64	21

Vulva and vagina operations

Study	Age	n	Deaths	%											
Bentzen and Anker (139)	70	75	2	2.7	1	–	–	1	1	–	–	–	–	–	–
Berger et al. (140)	60	328	7	2.1	–	2	2	1	–	–	–	–	–	1	1
Braitenberg (149)	70	?	1	?	–	2	1	–	–	–	–	–	–	–	–
Curiel and Morresi (159)	65	435	6	1.4	–	2	1	1	1	–	2	–	–	1	1
Douglas and Studdiford (167)	65	92	4	4.3	–	–	–	3	–	–	–	–	–	–	–
Fioretti and Andriani (171)	60	113	4	3.5	–	4	4	–	–	–	–	–	–	–	–
Kolářová and Staníček (206)	60	197	1	0.5	1	1	–	1	–	–	–	–	–	–	–
Lash (212)	60	244	8	3.3	–	1	–	–	3	1	2	–	–	–	–
Lucisano (225)	60	219	4	1.9	–	3	1	1	–	–	–	–	–	–	–
Maurizio and Pescetto (231)	60	38	1	2.6	–	–	1	–	–	–	–	–	–	–	–
Navratil (244)	65	267	7	2.6	–	5	1	1	–	–	–	–	1	1	1
O'Leary and Symmonds (250)	65	72	1	1.4	–	–	1	–	–	–	–	–	–	–	–
Piton (258)	65	65	1	1.5	–	–	–	–	–	–	–	–	–	–	–
Polito et al. (260)	60	168	1	0.6	–	1	1	–	–	–	–	–	–	–	–
Randow and Riess (263)	60	308	8	2.6	–	6	2	–	–	–	–	–	–	–	–
Rieppi et al. (266)	60	417	5	1.2	–	4	1	1	–	–	–	–	–	–	–
Rio (268)	60	59	1	1.6	–	–	1	–	–	–	1	–	–	–	–
Suonoja et al. (293)	60	331	1	0.3	–	1	–	–	–	–	–	–	–	–	–
Szendi and Lakatos (296)	60	262	1	0.4	–	–	–	–	–	–	1	–	–	–	–
Verrelli (311)	60	220	1	0.5	–	1	–	–	–	–	–	–	–	–	–
Total	–	–	65	–	2	28	13	8	5	1	5	–	1	1	2
Our material	60	2,782	58	2.1	3	24	5	4	6	4	4	–	1	1	7

Unknown nature of operation

Study	Age	n	Deaths	%											
Braitenberg (149)	70	?	8	?	–	4	1	–	–	–	–	–	–	2	2
Loskant (224)	60	?	2	?	–	1	–	1	–	–	–	–	–	1	–
Total	–	–	10	–	–	5	1	1	–	–	–	–	–	2	1

A relatively high percentage of women over 60 years old investigated as outpatients required inpatient treatment. Analysis of occupation of beds on gynecological wards gives us a better overview of the proportion of female geriatric patients in all inpatient admissions. From January 1st, 1973 to June 30th, 1973, 32.8% of the gynecological beds in our hospital were occupied by women who were 60 years old and older.

The proportion of old women in cancer preventive examinations is small. A 'low readiness to undergo examination' in these women and a middling interest of the gynecologist for the diseases of very old women may be the explanation for this. After popular lectures in old people's homes and social centers for seniors, there was a greater readiness to undergo gynecological examinations for cancer prevention. The intensification of the information talk should continue to be among our tasks.

More than 100 papers on surgical geriatric gynecology were analyzed. Only communications on a large material can contribute to solving the problems which still exist. Monothematic contributions on clinical problems of geriatric gynecology are becoming increasingly topical. Up to now, problems of geriatric gynecology have mostly been treated from the 60th year of life. This lower age limit will shift with increasing life expectancy. Subdivision of the operation material into age groups comprising 5 years therefore appears to be expedient.

The marked increase in geriatric patients undergoing surgery is to be explained by two factors: (1) more women reach the age and (2) the intensive and successful cooperation with other specialist disciplines during the entire treatment. All previous suggestions for estimation of the risk of surgery depend on subjective appraisal. Cooperation both with the internist and with the anesthetist is necessary for objective preoperative assessment of the risk of surgery. Small interventions may not be left out as up to now in the evaluation of surgical geriatric gynecology. Due attention was given to specific geriatric problems in the development of anesthesiology. In recent years, neuroleptic analgesia (which is especially suitable for laparotomy) has been added to the proved techniques of anesthesia.

The data in the literature enable the following classification of the kinds of diseases: malignant tumors, benign tumors, genital displacements and other diseases. In almost all communications, the genital displacements constituted the largest group. The often only global information in the literature permitted classification of the methods of surgery into only two groups: laparotomies and vaginal operations with operations on the vulva. We failed to find a differentiation of the laparotomies in the literature.

Consistent treatment of postoperative morbidity is becoming of growing significance. Besides general tasks, a specific evaluation of individual postoperative complications adapted to age is to be aimed for.

Postoperative mortality is one of the most important problems in surgical geriatric gynecology. A complete statistical registration without limitation is to be demanded. We account under postoperative lethality all cases which occurred during the stay in the hospital after an operation. Information on the carrying out or omission of an autopsy are rarely available. Information on the time of death and the age of the patients is often lacking. Diagnoses and data on the operations in patients who have died are also fragmentary. Many authors calculated a corrected mortality after subtraction of the deaths of women with malignancies. The immediate cause of death and not the fatal postoperative complication is frequently included in the statistics. Malignant tumors are by far the largest group of postoperative mortalities. This must be said to justify the extended indication for geriatric gynecological operations. We have noted pulmonary embolism as the most frequent cause of death; its preoperative and postoperative prophylaxis remains one of our most important tasks. In second place is cardiovascular failure. In the cases which were not autopsied, we can hardly recognize this diagnosis as a direct complication leading to death.

Special Chapter

General Analysis

In two West Berlin University Departments of Gynecology and Obstetrics and in 15 municipal hospitals, large operations had been undertaken on 7,151 60-year-old and older women in the years 1960–1969. 6,658 case records were registered and analyzed in a uniform manner by one person. Our operation material differed in this from the collected statistics already mentioned by *Vácha* (306). We conformed with regard to the mode of analysis to the specifications in the literature. Because of the varying extent of case history recording and the non-uniform description of the postoperative courses, we had to dispense with an analysis of the multimorbidity and postoperative complications.

Within the main research project fields of the Free University of Berlin 'Study of Statistics Systems', we were able to work with the Statistics Program SPSS (NORC) and the data computer IBM/360-67. This method of processing opened up new possibilities for complex analysis of numerous problems of clinical statistics in the geriatric gynecology. Of the combinations offered, merely the connections between kind of disease and mode of operations, as well as all factors of postoperative mortality are dealt with.

The following analysis, which is deliberately kept general, is intended to prove the clinical applicability of our conception of 'surgical geriatric gynecology'. In the following sections, a few case histories with atypical course will be mentioned. It is not intended to criticize the behavior of colleagues. On the contrary, we wish to demonstrate in this way the intricate clinical problems in surgical treatment of geriatric gynecological patients. We wish to point out possibilities of qualitative improvements.

Hospitals

The 17 gynecology departments participated to different extents in the overall operation material (e.g. department 0: 1,146 operations = 17.2%, and department 16: 72 operations = 1.1%). The 4,483 interventions make up 67.3%

of our material in the six largest gynecological wards. The three smallest departments, each with under 100 operations, have in the meantime been closed. A comparison of the departments reveals a differing attitude to individual techniques of surgery in the same disease and a quite dissimilar interest in carrying out autopsy of patients who have died postoperatively. The further differences are not significant. The material of individual departments was made available to us only for general analysis. For this reason, we refrain from further comparisons.

Age Groups

We have undertaken a classification into five 5-year groups. An appreciable age shift within the period investigated and in the two 5-year groups (1960– 1964 = 2,701 operations, 1965–1969 = 3,957 operations) cannot be detected. The absolute figures of the patients in all age groups are comparable with those in the literature. This also applies to the group of 261 women who were at least 80 years old, which is the best proof of the increasing clinical topicality of surgical geriatric gynecology (195). All further age-related data are found in the sections which follow.

Duration of Treatment

We used the data at the top of the patient record to register the duration of treatment. The investigation thus also includes interim stays in other wards before and after the intervention. The recorded duration of treatment is longer than known from the literature. An overview is provided by the following tables. In our 6,658 cases, the duration of treatment was on average 40.6 days. The preoperative preparation lasted 9.8 days and the postoperative care 30.8 days. The duration of inpatient treatment depends on many factors, so that a general analysis is of limited value. The data obtained by electronic data processing can, however, contribute to the analysis of individual problems in geriatric gynecology.

Kind of Operation

Prior analysis of the surgical methods applied enables us to incorporate these later with the individual diseases in a complex consideration. For better registration of the multiplicity of surgical techniques, we have in contrast to the

Table 35. Age groups, average age and duration of treatment in operation groups

Operation group	Total cases	Age groups, years										Average age	Average duration of treatment, days		
		60–64		65–69		70–74		75–79		80 and over		age years	total	before operation	after operation
		n	%	n	%	n	%	n	%	n	%				
Vulva operations	121	23	19.0	29	24.0	37	30.6	21	17.4	11	9.1	70.6	49.8	9.8	40.0
Vaginal operations on the descensus	1,174	509	43.4	386	32.9	191	16.3	77	6.6	11	0.9	66.2	30.8	7.5	23.3
Vaginal operations on uterine prolapse	695	166	23.9	193	27.8	200	28.8	89	12.8	47	6.8	69.6	34.8	9.4	25.4
Abdomino-vaginal descensus/ prolapse operations	124	65	52.4	43	34.7	12	9.7	3	2.4	1	0.8	65.0	34.8	6.9	27.9
Vaginal operations	468	201	42.9	120	25.6	101	21.6	33	7.1	13	2.8	66.9	45.0	12.4	32.6
'Total' gynecological laparotomies	2,042	759	37.2	653	32.0	394	19.3	185	9.0	51	2.5	67.3	41.1	10.6	30.5
Gynecological palliative, exploratory, and emergency laparotomies	621	222	35.7	183	29.5	118	19.0	70	11.3	28	4.5	67.9	46.7	13.2	33.5
'Total' surgical laparotomies	171	73	42.7	44	25.7	25	14.6	19	11.1	10	5.8	67.7	38.6	9.6	29.0
Surgical palliative, exploratory, and emergency laparotomies	117	33	28.2	35	29.9	34	29.1	10	8.5	5	4.3	68.2	43.5	12.0	31.5
Breast operations	1,125	326	29.0	318	28.3	251	22.3	146	13.0	84	7.5	69.0	47.8	8.4	39.4
Total	6,658	2,377	35.7	2,004	30.1	1,363	20.5	653	9.8	261	3.9	67.7	40.6	9.8	30.8

literature extended their classification (table 35). The following tables show that thanks to the large amount of material available to us the analysis of the kinds of operation with 'additional interventions' has yielded clinically useful insights.

Vulva Operations

In the 121 vulva operations, a hemivulvectomy was more frequently involved than an ablatio vulvae. In some operation records we have noticed an unusual nomenclature in vulva operations: bilateral vulvectomy (676/0), subtotal vulvectomy (882/0), partial hemivulvectomy (424/2).

We suggested the following classification of operations on the vulva: (1) radical vulvectomy, (2) vulvectomy, (3) hemivulvectomy, (4) tumor extirpation, (5) exploratory excision, and (6) other vulva operations (e.g. Burger, Horn, Mering operations etc.).

Operations on Genital Displacements

We list the crucial phases of the 1,869 vaginal operations in genital descensus and prolapsus with the additional interventions in table 36. The methods of operation were greatly dependent on the department and in some cases age-dependent.

The 205 portio amputations were mainly carried out according to the technique of Fothergill. In the group 'anterior and posterior colporrhaphy', posterior colporrhaphy was mostly involved, carried out in the sense of a 'colpocleisis'. The reasons for dispensing with operation on the anterior wall of the vagina cannot be traced retrospectively. Labhardt semicolpocleisis and posterior colporrhaphy (often termed as 'high') are qualitatively comparable.

The 52 cases of a Schauta-Wertheim uterine interposition constitutes only 2.6% of all descensus and prolapsus operations. In our view, this intervention is no longer to be regarded as a modern surgical technique.

The number of adnexae removed along with vaginal hysterectomies and vaginal stump extirpations is small. In view of increasing life expectancy, bilateral salpingo-oophorectomy should already be considered as 'oncological geroprophylaxis' in women in early and late postmenopause and dispensing with this intervention should only be accepted in exceptional cases.

We regard that all corrections of genital displacements by laparotomy are an inappropriate intervention in descensus conditions of old women. We should therefore like to give the 124 'abdominal' or 'abdominovaginal' operations of descensus or prolapsus vaginae et uteri an especially thorough analysis (table 37).

Table 36. Vaginal operation on genital displacements

Crucial phase of operation	Cases n	Cases %	Additional intervention none	with colporrhaphies, without adnexae	without colporrhaphies, without adnexae	with colporrhaphies, with adnexae	without colporrhaphies, with adnexae	Labhardt's operation	posterior colporrhaphy	Neugebauer-LeFort's operation	other operations
Vaginal hysterectomy	419	22.4	–	351	8	33	4	19	–	3	1
Vaginal stump extirpation	32	1.7	–	27	1	–	–	4	1	–	–
Portio amputation	205	11.0	–	192	1	–	–	9	1	2	–
Anterior and posterior colporrhaphies	495	26.5	495	–	–	–	–	–	–	–	–
Anterior or posterior colporrhaphy	137	7.3	96	–	–	–	–	41	–	–	–
Conill's operation	28	1.5	28	–	–	–	–	–	–	–	–
Uterine interposition	52	2.8	8	–	–	–	–	2	41	1	–
Labhardt's operation	243	13.0	241	1	–	–	–	–	–	–	1
Neugebauer-LeFort's operation	215	11.5	20	–	–	–	–	85	99	–	1
Döderlein's operation	16	0.9	7	–	–	–	–	1	8	–	–
Other operations	27	1.4	23	–	–	–	–	–	4	–	–
Total	1,869	100.0	918	571	9	33	4	171	154	6	3

Table 37. Abdominal and abdominovaginal operations of genital displacements

Kind of operation	Total cases			Descensus cases			Prolapse cases		
	n	also vaginal	only abdominal	n	also vaginal	only abdominal	n	also vaginal	only abdominal
Abdominal hysterectomy	11	6	5	6	1	5	5	5	–
Abdominal stump extirpation	2	1	1	2	1	1	–	–	–
Alexander-Adams' operation	42	39	3	41	38	3	1	1	–
Doléris' operation or Kocher's operation	22	6	16	13	5	8	9	1	8
Marshall-Marchetti's operation	27	5	22	27	5	22	–	–	–
Bracht's operation	8	6	2	8	6	2	–	–	–
Other operations	12	6	6	4	2	2	8	4	4
Total	124	69	55	101	58	43	23	11	12

The 'abdominal operations' were combined 69 times (55.6%) with a vaginal intervention. The vaginal intervention was omitted 55 times (44.4%). Table 37 shows that in a women's hospital the uterus was prefixed 42 times according to Alexander-Adams (39 times with vaginal colporrhaphies). These also include the 8 cases of restraining colporrhaphy according to Bracht and 27 Marshall-Marchetti operations. The last kind of operation was only combined 4 times with a colporrhaphy. One can thus assume that in the majority of the women the urinary incontinence without the anatomical finding typical for a descensus or prolapsus was the main indication for surgery. The 11 abdominal hysterectomies and the 2 abdominal stump extirpations can be considered as fully fledged descensus or prolapsus operations. There thus remain 22 Doléris antefixation operations or Kocher exohysteropexies. These constitute 1.1% of all operations on genital displacements and are to be designated as department-associated.

Here some examples of operations which we regard as outmoded:

Case 371/0: Total prolapse of cervix. Doléris ventrofixation of the stump.
Case 404/0: Total prolapse. Supravaginal uterine amputation and adnectomy on the right. Fixation of the stump to the symphysis plus posterior colporrhaphy.
Case 937/1: Uterus myomatosus and descensus vaginae. 'Since an anterior and posterior colporrhaphy is necessary in the patient, the uterus will by way of exception be amputated supravaginally.' No fixation of the vagina to the round ligaments.
Case 29/11: Decubitus on the prolapsed uterine stump. PE: Carcinoma in situ, three radium applications with a total of 4,000 mgeh; afterwards stump fixation to the abdominal rectus muscles.

Table 38. Vaginal operations

Crucial phase of operation	Cases		Additional intervention				
	n	%	with colpor-rhaphies, without adnexae	without colpor-rhaphies, without adnexae	with colpor-rhaphies, with adnexae	without colpor-rhaphies, with adnexae	none
Schauta's operation	104	22.2	4	79	2	19	–
Vaginal hysterectomy	308	65.8	13	128	12	155	–
Vaginal stump extirpation	13	2.8	2	8	–	3	–
Fistula operation	23	4.9	–	–	–	–	23
Other vaginal operations	20	4.3	5	–	–	5	10
Total	468	100.0	24	215	14	182	33

Case 148/11: Total prolapse. Supravaginal uterine amputation with stump fixation to the abdominal wall.

Case 18/14: Total prolapse. Although a hydrometra is described in the surgical record, a ventrofixatio uteri was carried out.

Vaginal Operations

We have listed 468 vaginal operations in the treatment of malignant and benign tumors as well as other gynecological diseases (table 38). If small operations were taken into account, this group would greatly increase in size.

Laparotomies

The classification into gynecological and surgical laparotomies which we selected is to be seen from table 39. We further subdivide into operations with complete or with incomplete removal of the organ concerned.

'Complete gynecological laparotomies' are registered in table 40 and with the supplementary operations in table 41. We have also assigned the supravaginal uterine amputations and the salpingo-oophorectomies in benign tumors here. Nevertheless, we believe that abdominal hysterectomy with removal of the adnexae is to be regarded as the method of choice. For this reason, one cannot designate a hysterectomy in which the adnexae are left in place as a complete operation even in geriatric patients with benign tumors (the same applies for simple abdominal or vaginal stump extirpation in a collum carcinoma).

Table 39. Age groups, average age and duration of treatment in different kinds of laparotomy

Kind of laparotomy	Total cases	Age groups, years										Average age, years	Average duration of treatment, days		
		60–64		65–69		70–74		75–79		80 and over			total	before operation	after operation
		n	%	n	%	n	%	n	%	n	%				
'Complete' gynecological laparotomies	2,042	759	37.2	653	32.0	394	19.3	185	9.0	51	2.5	67.3	41.1	10.6	30.5
Gynecological palliative laparotomies	297	103	34.7	83	27.9	57	19.2	36	12.1	18	6.1	68.3	47.2	11.7	35.5
Gynecological exploratory laparotomies	249	91	36.5	78	31.3	47	18.9	26	10.4	7	2.8	67.7	42.0	12.5	29.5
Gynecological emergency laparotomies	75	28	37.3	22	29.3	14	18.7	8	10.7	3	4.0	67.3	60.6	21.4	39.2
'Complete' surgical laparotomies	171	73	42.7	44	25.7	25	14.6	19	11.1	10	5.8	67.7	38.6	9.6	29.0
Surgical palliative laparotomies	12	4	33.3	7	58.4	–	–	1	8.3	–	–	66.2	53.0	9.9	43.1
Surgical exploratory laparotomies	88	24	27.2	25	28.4	28	31.9	7	8.0	4	4.5	68.4	43.3	12.8	30.5
Surgical emergency laparotomies	17	5	29.4	3	17.6	6	35.8	2	11.8	1	5.9	68.5	37.3	9.1	28.2
Total laparotomies	2,951	1,087	36.8	915	31.0	571	19.3	284	9.6	94	3.3	67.4	42.1	11.1	31.0
Total interventions	6,658	2,377	35.7	2,004	30.1	1,363	20.5	653	9.8	261	3.9	67.7	40.6	9.8	30.8

Table 40. Age groups, average age and duration of treatment in 'complete' gynecological laparotomies

'Complete' gynecological laparotomies	Total cases	Age groups, years										Average age	Average duration of treatment, days		
		60–64		65–69		70–74		75–79		80 and over		age years	total	before operation	after operation
		n	%	n	%	n	%	n	%	n	%				
Wertheim's operation	118	66	55.9	45	38.1	6	5.1	1	0.8	–	–	64.2	66.4	17.3	49.1
Hysterectomy	1,248	490	39.3	412	33.0	215	17.2	103	8.3	28	2.2	67.0	41.8	10.6	31.2
Supravaginal uterine amputation	100	26	26.0	36	36.0	25	25.0	13	13.0	–	–	68.1	39.2	10.1	29.1
Stump extirpation	12	8	66.7	4	33.3	–	–	–	–	–	–	63.4	34.9	10.3	24.6
Unilateral salpingo-cophorectomy	412	118	28.6	111	26.9	115	27.9	49	11.9	19	4.6	68.7	33.6	8.8	24.8
Bilateral salpingo-oophorectomy	114	33	28.9	35	30.7	26	22.8	16	14.0	4	3.5	68.8	33.9	8.7	25.2
Myoma enucleation	16	4	25.0	5	31.3	4	25.0	3	18.7	–	–	68.8	31.7	9.4	22.4
Adhesiolysis	6	4	66.7	2	33.3	–	–	–	–	–	–	63.5	31.5	12.0	19.5
Fistula operations	11	6	54.5	3	27.3	2	18.2	–	–	–	–	65.0	69.2	18.9	50.3
Other laparotomies	5	4	80.0	–	–	1	20.0	–	–	–	–	65.0	58.0	18.6	39.4
Total	2,042	759	37.2	653	32.0	394	19.3	185	9.0	51	2.5	67.3	41.1	10.6	30.5
Total interventions	6,658	2,377	35.7	2,004	30.1	1,363	20.5	653	9.8	261	3.9	67.7	40.6	9.8	30.8

Table 41. 'Complete'gynecological laparotomies and additional operations

Crucial phase of operation	Cases		Additional intervention				
	n	%	2 adnexae, 2 removed	2 adnexae, 1 removed	2 adnexae, none removed	1 adnexa, 1 removed	none
Wertheim's operation or evisceration	118	5.8	117	–	1	–	–
Abdominal hysterectomy	1,248	61.1	1,182	2	13[1]	46	5[2]
Supravaginal uterine amputation	100	4.9	53	21	20	6	–
Abdominal stump extirpation	12	0.6	4	–	–	8	–
Unilateral salpingo-oophorectomy	412	20.2	–	403	–	9	–
Bilateral salpingo-oophorectomy	114	5.6	114	–	–	–	–
Myoma enucleation	16	0.8	4	1	11	–	–
Adhesiolysis	6	0.3	–	–	–	–	6
Fistula operations	11	0.5	1	–	–	–	10
Other operations	5	0.2	–	–	–	–	5
Total	2,042	100.0	1,475	427	45	69	26

[1] One adnexa present in 1 case and not removed.
[2] No adnexae in 5 cases.

In our 297 palliative gynecological operations, a tumor extirpation was involved 66 times, the removal of both adnexae in ovarian malignancies 64 times, unilateral salpingo-oophorectomy in ovarian cancer in 75 cases, and a supravaginal uterine amputation with or without adnexae 73 times (table 42). The clinical problems of the 249 gynecological experimental laparotomies has in the meantime been treated in a separate communication (196).

In 75 gynecological emergency laparotomies, an anus praeter naturalis was applied 63 times and an intestinal fistula 8 times; a drainage of the abdomen was performed twice and ureter implantation twice. These figures have only limited reliability, since many emergency laparotomies in gynecological malignancies were carried out in surgery departments.

The 171 'complete surgical operations' involved 39 appendectomies, 47 colon resections, 7 small intestinal resections, 25 scar hernias, and 9 other hernias. The 44 'other operations' comprised 33 exclusively gynecological operations on a surgical condition (13 malignant tumors, 10 benign tumors and 10 sigmoid diverticulitis cases) as well as 11 small surgical interventions in rare pathological findings. In the meantime, we have analyzed 88 exploratory surgical laparotomies (196). We shall not go into details of the 12 palliative surgical laparotomies and 17 emergency surgical laparotomies.

Breast Operations

A remarkably divergent designation of the same interventions is to be noted in the registration of the 1,125 breast operations. In contrast to other gynecological operations, the operations specified in the surgical record thus cannot simply be taken over.

Kind of Diseases

In contrast to the literature, we subdivided our 6,658 patients into five groups according to the kind of disease. In table 43 we combine all diseases with age groups, average age and duration of treatment.

Genital Displacements

In the literature, the genital displacements mostly constituted the largest group of diseases. Our 1,993 cases constitute only 29.9% of the entire surgical material. Both in descensus and in prolapse patients we have used a classification which is not yet usual in the geriatric literature: (1) women with uterus, (2) women with cervical stump, and (3) women with blindly ending vagina (table 44). Despite the anatomical differences, descensus and prolapse patients are analyzed together (table 45). In 1,759 women (88.3%) it was the first operation and in 234 (11.7%) it was a relapse operation. The descensus patients operated on were on average 66.1 years old; the prolapse patients were 3.5 years older, i.e. 69.6 years old.

The proportion of genital displacements (particularly descensus) in the entire patient material continuously decreases with increasing age. Two conclusions can be drawn from this fact:

(1) Anomalies in the position of the female genitals cannot be assigned exclusively to the geriatric patients. Surgical treatment should not be delayed too long.

(2) A descensus and in particular a prolapse of the uterus, the portio or the blindly ending vagina have not lost their significance for surgical geriatric gynecology.

Table 42. Palliative operations in some malignancies

Kind of palliative laparotomy	Total cases	Uterine cervix	Corpus uteri	Tube	Ovary	General carcinosis
Tumor extirpation	66	3	10	2	51	–
Salpingo-oophorectomy, bilateral	64	–	–	1	63	–
Salpingo-oophorectomy, unilateral (2 adnexae present)	75	–	–	3	71	1
Salpingo-oophorectomy, unilateral (1 adnexa present)	5	–	–	–	4	1
Supravaginal uterine amputation with adnexae	72	6	16	2	47	1
Supravaginal uterine amputation without adnexae	1	–	1	–	–	–
Vaginal stump extirpation	11	9	2	–	–	–
Abdominal stump extirpation	3	3	–	–	–	–
Total	297	21	29	8	236	3

Many papers have been published on the advantages of surgical treatment of genital displacements. A medical indication for pessary treatment is only rarely present today. It would be in the interest of the patients if the colleagues in free practises were to share this view. The number of pessary wearers registered by the health insurance schemes is still very great. The elimination of this medically unjustifiable practise should be seen as a measure for prevention of geriatric gynecological illnesses.

We have already commented on individual surgical techniques, so that we only make a few remarks here:

(1) Antefixation operations are becoming increasingly rare. The advantages of the Fothergill operation are generally known. However, they become effective practically only in younger women. In geriatric patients, this operation cannot be counted as a standard operation since the corpus uteri and the adnexae are left in place.

Colporrhaphies serve solely to eliminate the descensus vaginae with cystocele and rectocele and are not suitable for dealing with descensus uteri. On the other hand, besides the elimination of the symptoms connected with the

Table 43. Age groups, average age and duration of treatment in the diagnosis groups

Diagnosis group	Total cases	Age groups, years										Average age, years	Average duration of treatment, days		
		60–64		65–69		70–74		75–79		80 and over			total	before operation	after operation
		n	%	n	%	n	%	n	%	n	%				
Genital displacements	1,993	740	37.1	622	31.2	403	20.2	169	8.5	59	3.0	67.3	32.6	8.3	24.3
Malignant tumors	3,111	1,042	33.5	965	30.4	638	20.5	331	10.6	155	5.0	68.1	48.0	11.0	37.0
Benign tumors	1,141	389	34.1	330	28.9	271	23.8	115	10.1	36	3.2	67.9	35.0	8.9	26.1
Other gynecological diseases	266	137	51.5	72	27.1	32	12.0	21	7.9	4	1.5	65.9	40.1	12.5	27.6
Other surgical diseases	147	69	46.9	35	23.8	19	12.9	17	11.6	7	4.8	67.2	34.8	8.6	26.2
Total	6,658	2,377	35.7	2,004	30.1	1,364	20.5	653	9.8	261	3.9	67.7	40.6	9.8	30.8

Table 44. Age groups, average age and duration of treatment in genital displacements

Genital displacement	Total cases	Age groups, years										Aver- age	Average duration of treatment, days		
		60–64		65–69		70–74		75–79		80 and over		age years	total	be- fore oper- ation	after oper- ation
		n	%	n	%	n	%	n	%	n	%				
Uterine descensus	1,203	530	44.1	398	33.1	189	15.7	76	6.3	10	0.8	66.1	30.9	7.6	23.3
Descensus of cervix stump	39	23	59.0	12	30.8	3	7.7	1	2.6	–	–	64.7	30.7	6.8	23.9
Descensus of blindly ending vagina	33	14	42.4	11	33.3	6	18.2	1	3.0	1	3.0	66.1	35.9	9.3	26.6
Uterine prolapse	665	159	23.9	180	27.1	195	29.3	84	12.6	47	7.1	69.7	35.4	9.5	25.9
Prolapse of cervix stump	30	8	26.7	11	36.7	7	23.3	4	13.3	–	–	68.2	38.5	9.8	28.7
Prolapse of blindly ending vagina	23	6	26.1	10	43.5	3	13.0	1	4.3	1	4.3	67.8	31.5	6.9	24.6
Total	1,993	740	37.1	622	31.2	403	20.2	169	8.5	59	3.0	67.3	32.6	8.3	24.3
Total cases	6,658	2,377	35.7	2,004	30.1	1,363	20.5	683	9.8	261	3.9	67.7	40.6	9.8	30.8

Table 45. Crucial phases of genital displacement operations

Crucial phase of operation	Total cases	Descensus			Prolapse		
		uterus	cervix stump	only vagina	uterus	cervix stump	only vagina
Vaginal hysterectomy	419	198	–	–	221	–	–
Vaginal stump extirpation	32	–	20	–	–	12	–
Portio amputation	205	174	–	–	31	–	–
Anterior and posterior colporrhaphies	495	418	10	20	36	4	7
Anterior or posterior colporrhaphy	137	129	2	6	–	–	–
Uterine interposition	52	29	–	–	23	–	–
Labhardt's operation	243	101	1	5	126	3	7
Neugebauer-Le Fort's operation	215	39	1	–	163	8	4
Conill's operation	28	–	–	–	27	–	1
Döderlein's operation	16	–	–	–	16	–	–
Abdominal hysterectomy	11	6	–	–	5	–	–
Alexander-Adams' operation	42	41	–	–	1	–	–
Doléris' operation or Kocher's operation	22	13	–	–	8	1	–
Marshall-Marchetti's operation	27	27	–	–	–	–	–
Other operations	49	28	5	2	8	2	4
Total	1,993	1,203	39	33	665	30	23

descensus or prolapsus uteri, hysterectomy enables at the same time an effective prophylaxis of geriatric gynecological diseases.

Vaginal hysterectomy with colporrhaphies has logically developed to become the method of choice in the treatment of genital displacements. *Berle et al.* (141) as well as *Kindermann* (204) point out a change from palliative to irrevocable surgical techniques in descensus and prolapse of the genitals. This tendency is clearly manifested in our material. If one divides the period investigated into 5-year intervals, a slight rise (1960–1964: 13.6%; 1965–1969: 19.3%) is shown in the treatment of descensus patients, and a marked increase of vaginal hysterectomy is shown in prolapse patients (1960–1964: 23.6%; 1965–1969: 38.0%). The difference between the years 1960 (16.7%) and 1969 (46.9%) is still greater. The broader indication for vaginal hysterectomy in elderly prolapse patients today encounters a gratifying openmindedness on the part of the patients, who are frequently interested in an active lovelife in old age.

Besides this, the vaginal closure operations have not lost clinical importance. Although many modifications are known, we were able to observe in the material of the West Berlin gynecology departments almost exclusively Neugebauer-Le Fort semicolpocleisis in combination with Labhardt's operation or a 'high' posterior colporrhaphy (91.2% of all semicolpocleises). The Döderlein operation has not attained very great popularity. Its use was clearly department-associated. With the Conill operation, relapses were often observed; this corresponds with our own experience.

In our view, vaginal hysterectomy with colporrhaphies, Labhardt's semicolpocleisis or colpohysterectomy are also gaining increasing significance in elderly women who are no longer sexually active.

(2) It would be welcomed if genital displacements were less frequently the reason for surgical intervention in elderly women. The ratio between descensus and prolapse should be changed in favor of vaginal descensus. This might be interpreted as a sign of timely operation.

Some shifts are to be expected within the three groups which we formed. The fewer supravaginal uterine amputations are performed, the more rarely will cases of descensus or prolapse of the portio stump occur. Another development is to be expected in descensus or prolapse of the blindly ending vagina. This possibility should have been thought of even at the first intervention, i.e. in vaginal or abdominal hysterectomy. In our view, this operation should include suturing of both round ligaments with the base of the vagina. This small intervention can be seen as a measure for prevention of later descensus symptoms. In 20 cases of descensus or prolapse after prior hysterectomy or supravaginal uterine amputation, the end of the vagina or the portio stump is not attached to the round ligament.

(3) The number of abrasions in isolated colporrhaphies is surprisingly small. Even in a semicolpocleisis, a fractionated abrasion is not always carried out. We should like to point out the necessity of preoperative diagnostics before prolapse operations with some examples.

Case 924/1: 6 months previously a Neugebauer-Le Fort operation without abrasion. Abrasion through the right, relatively broad vaginal canal because of hemorrhages. Histology: corpus carcinoma; therapy: vaginal hysterectomy with adnexae and colporrhaphies.

Case 541/1: Despite reported smear bleeding, no PAP smear and no abrasion, but the same Neugebauer-Le Fort operation with 'high' posterior colporrhaphy. After 1 year, an abdominal hysterectomy was necessary because of recurrent hemorrhage. In the cavum uteri, a large corpus polyp was found.

Case 57/10: Total uterine prolapse, vaginal hysterectomy without adnexae, collum carcinoma as a chance finding.

Case 333/2: Descensus vaginae et uteri. No abrasion, vaginal hysterectomy without adnexae. Histology: carcinoma corporis uteri.

Case 222/12: Descensus vaginae et uteri. Anterior and posterior colporrhaphy with Manchester's operation. Histology: carcinoma in situ.

Table 46. Age groups, average age and duration of treatment in malignancies

Localization of malignancy	Total cases	Age groups, years										Average age, years	Average duration of treatment, days		
		60–64		65–69		70–74		75–79		80 and over			total	before operation	after operation
		n	%	n	%	n	%	n	%	n	%				
Vulva	87	10	11.5	20	23.0	32	36.8	16	18.4	9	10.3	71.5	57.4	10.7	46.7
Vagina	15	2	13.3	4	26.7	4	26.7	3	20.0	2	13.3	71.9	50.0	12.5	38.5
Uterine cervix	326	167	51.2	112	34.4	32	9.8	12	3.7	3	0.9	65.1	61.0	16.1	44.9
Corpus uteri	763	279	36.6	233	30.5	156	20.5	72	9.4	23	3.0	67.5	44.0	12.5	31.5
Tube	29	8	27.6	14	48.3	6	20.7	1	3.4	–	–	67.1	48.2	9.4	35.8
Ovary	604	206	34.1	190	31.5	116	19.2	69	11.4	23	3.8	67.9	46.2	11.1	35.1
General carcinosis	37	13	31.9	12	31.9	6	19.1	2	6.4	4	10.6	68.7	39.8	13.5	26.3
Extragenital intraperitoneal malignancy	106	27	26.0	32	31.0	30	27.0	10	10.0	7	6.0	69.0	46.1	6.6	39.5
Extraperitoneal malignancy	19	4	21.1	10	52.6	5	26.3	–	–	–	–	67.1	57.0	23.8	33.2
Breast	1,125	326	29.0	318	28.3	251	22.3	146	13.0	84	7.5	69.0	47.6	2.8	44.8
Total	3,111	1,042	33.5	945	30.4	638	20.5	331	10.6	155	5.0	68.1	48.0	11.0	37.0
Total cases	6,658	2,377	35.7	2,004	30.1	1,363	20.5	653	9.8	261	3.9	67.7	40.6	9.8	30.8

It is wrong not to wait for histological clarification in macroscopically or cytologically suspect findings:

Case 484/0: Because of a suspect portio, an exploratory excision was made and a Neugebauer-Le Fort semicolpocleisis was carried out immediately afterwards. The histological examination revealed a collum carcinoma. The 79-year-old patient was then merely irradiated with the betatron.

Worthy of mention in addition is case 429/3: In a patient with prolapse recurrence the uterus was perforated in an abrasion. An abdominal hysterectomy with both adnexae and an operation according to Labhardt were carried out. The correctness of also removing the adnexae, in uterine extirpations after the menopause, was confirmed by the histology, which revealed a papillary carcinoma *in situ* in the right tube.

Among the patients with a corpus carcinoma, we found 4 with a total prolapse in whom the malignancy was diagnosed by an abrasion before the operation (179/5, 12/9, 478/4, 294/4).

Malignant Tumors

The 3,111 malignant tumors operated on constitute 46.7% of the total material (table 46). In contrast to data in the literature, they constitute the largest group of diseases in our surgical material. The consideration of mammary carcinomas contributes to this but even without them, the proportion of malignancies would be relatively high with us.

Vulvar Carcinoma

Vulvar carcinoma is a typical geriatric malignancy. Actinotherapy is often preferred for its treatment. The 87 cases which were operated on are not representative for the frequency of vulvar carcinoma. They constitute merely 2.8% of all malignancies operated on. For this reason, a statistical breakdown is dispensed with here.

Carcinoma of the Vagina

Vaginal carcinoma is difficult to deal with surgically and primary radiation is performed in the majority of cases. We are therefore able to report on only 15 operations on histologically verified vaginal carcinomas from six women's hospitals; 4 radical operations were undertaken (1 abdominal and 1 vaginal hysterectomy with vaginal cuff), there were 6 tumor extirpations and an anus praeter was applied 3 times.

Collum Carcinoma

Table 47 gives a survey of the interventions in 326 collum carcinomas. After examination of the surgical records, we have assigned 5 operations to the vaginal hysterectomies because they had been inappropriately designated as radical vaginal uterine extirpations.

Table 47. Kind of operation in some malignancies

Kind of operation	Total		Uterine cervix		Corpus uteri		Tube		Ovary		General carcinosis	
	n	%	n	%	n	%	n	%	n	%	n	%
Schauta's operation	103	5.9	97	29.8	6	0.8	–	–	–	–	–	–
Vaginal hysterectomy	228	13.0	19	5.8	208	27.2	1	3.4	–	–	–	–
Wertheim's operation	117	6.7	108[1]	33.1	6[2]	0.8	1	3.4	2[2]	0.3	–	–
Abdominal hysterectomy	722	40.9	38	11.7	477	62.5	12	41.4	191	31.6	4	10.8
Palliative operation	297	16.9	21	6.4	29	3.8	8	27.7	236	39.1	3	8.1
Exploratory laparotomy	231	13.1	10	3.1	30	3.9	7	24.1	156	25.9	28	75.7
Emergency laparotomy	61	3.5	33	10.1	7	0.9	–	–	19	3.1	2	5.4
Total	1,759	100.0	326	100.0	763	100.0	29	100.0	604	100.0	37	100.0

[1] One evisceration.
[2] Two eviscerations.

Radical Operations

Of 205 radical operations, 144 were carried out in three gynecology departments, a further 48 in four other gynecology departments and 13 in the rest of the gynecology departments. The varying attitude to vaginal and abdominal procedure is noteworthy: department 0 (52 Schauta, 4 Wertheim), department 1 (30 Schauta, 14 Wertheim) and department 2 (2 Schauta, 42 Wertheim). In the other departments, the Wertheim operation was preferred. In the 108 Wertheim operations, the adnexae were left in place in only 1 case. The situation is completely different in the 97 radical vaginal hysterectomies although the same malignancy was being treated. The adnexae had not been removed 82 times (84.5%).

We do not understand this procedure. The Schauta operation is reserved for the most experienced surgeon for whom removal of the adnexae does not constitute a technical problem. Even if one may perhaps be able to dispense with postoperative irradiation in a few favorable cases, the senile ovaries and tubes do not constitute a functional organ. This is not altered even by metastases of the collum carcinomas preferentially into the parametria.

Incomplete Operations

78 interventions can be designated as palliative and (especially in collum carcinoma) as incomplete. After subtraction of 3 'tumor extirpations' and 6 supravaginal uterine amputations, neither the 19 vaginal and 38 abdominal hysterectomies nor the 9 vaginal and 3 abdominal stump extirpations can be regarded as complete operations. The palliative operations can be subdivided into two groups.

Group 1: Collum carcinoma was known before intervention.

(a) The palliative operation was regarded as an adequate intervention. These include in the first incidence the vaginal hysterectomies already mentioned, which the surgeons designated as radical interventions. We found inconsistent thinking, e.g. in the following cases:

Case 85/15: 'After diagnosing a carcinoma of the neck of the uterus, the pathologist has suggested a portio amputation in the 64-year-old patient. In his opinion, a radical operation was not necessary. Since the parametria were free, we left the adnexae in on the advice of the pathologist.'

Case 566/02: 'On admission, the parametria were free and the internal genitals corresponded to the age.' Abdominal hysterectomy with adnexae.

Case 150/9: Collum carcinoma II, suspicion of pyometra. 'In view of the age of the patient (70 years) and since a radium irradiation was not indicated because of the pyometra, an abdominal hysterectomy with both adnexae was carried out.' The patient died 3 months later.

Case 99/2: 'In view of the general condition of the patient and the tendency to fall in blood pressure, radical surgery is refrained from and only an abdominal hysterectomy without adnexae is carried out.'

Case 58/6: 'A radical Wertheim operation was dispensed with because of the age (60 years) after no lymph nodes had been palpated in the small pelvis.'

Case 242/8: 'Because of obesity and the presenile state, merely an abdominal hysterectomy with both adnexae.'

(b) Palliative operations in non-indicated interventions.

Case 120/07: Collum carcinoma IV. Lymph node metastases in the small pelvis. Irradiation does not appear appropriate because of the extent of the tumor. In poor general condition, only abdominal hysterectomy with adnexae and lymph node extirpation.

Case 266/8: Collum carcinoma III. Wertheim not possible. Abdominal hysterectomy with both adnexae.

Case 95/8: Collum carcinoma III. As palliative operation, abdominal hysterectomy with adnexae.

Case 23/8: Collum carcinoma III–IV. Wertheim not technically possible. Abdominal hysterectomy with adnexae.

Case 378/4: Admission in a highly reduced and neglected general condition. Laparotomy. The collum carcinoma was so advanced that a radical operation was no longer possible. Therefore only a supravaginal uterine amputation with both adnexae (!).

Case 83/4: Preirradiated collum carcinoma with hydrometra. Supravaginal uterine amputation with both adnexae. The portio had to be left in place because of substantial adhesions with the bladder and the rectum.

(c) Palliative operations in previously irradiated cases.

Cases 237/4 vaginal stump extirpation, 516/4 vaginal stump extirpation, 158/4, 50/11 and 297/4 each abdominal hysterectomies with both adnexae.

Group 2: Collum carcinoma was not known before intervention.

These include some case histories in which we have not found any information on the preoperative diagnostics (cytological smear, fractional abrasion, exploratory excision or conization), and in which the diagnosis collum carcinoma had only been made during the histological examination of the surgical preparation. Cases 58/2, 178/4 and 7/11: abrasion material (without fractionated abrasion): microscopically, carcinoma of the body of the uterus or adenocarcinoma. Abdominal hysterectomy with adnexae. Histology: collum carcinoma.

In some cases (413/2, 297/5, 326/5, 395/5, 487/5) an operation was performed immediately because of suspect smears (portio amputation plus colporrhaphies, vaginal stump extirpation plus colporrhaphies, 3 vaginal hysterectomies without adnexae). A collum carcinoma was involved 4 times and there was an unequivocally benign finding in 1 case.

Case 484/0: Suspect erosion in total prolapse of the uterus. Exploratory excision and immediately afterwards a Neugebauer-Le Fort semicolpocleisis. A collum carcinoma was verified histologically and the patient was only irradiated percutaneously.

Case 116/8: Conization plus abrasion, unclear histology, therefore further clarification recommended. However, abdominal hysterectomy was performed immediately. The repeated histological examination revealed a collum carcinoma.

Case 138/4: Preoperative diagnosis pyometra. On laparotomy, 2,000 ml of pus were removed and the uterus therefore drained to the fornix. Collum carcinoma was not diagnosed. Exitus 4 months later. On autopsy, an advanced collum carcinoma.

Case 113/4: An abdominal hysterectomy was performed in the patient because of the diagnosis 'myoma submucosa necroticans'. It was in fact an advanced collum carcinoma.

Case 72/11: Recurrent bleeding in the postmenopause, descensus vaginae. No abrasion, no conization. Immediate vaginal hysterectomy without adnexae with colporrhaphy. Histology: carcinoma of the neck of the uterus.

Case 304/0: Brownish discharge, no abrasion. The patient has been operated on after diagnosis of a uterus myomatosus. Histology: 'In the collum is found an extensive infiltratively growing squamous epithelial carcinoma'.

Case 25/15: Suspicion of an ovarian tumor. Abdominal hysterectomy with both adnexae. Histology: Benign ovarian tumor on both sides and squamous epithelial carcinoma of the collum as a random finding.

Case 57/10: A total prolapse with 'decubital ulcer' and erosion. No smear, no exploratory excision. Vaginal hysterectomy without adnexae with colporrhaphy. Histology: Carcinoma of the neck of the uterus.

Case 412/2: Ovarian tumor on the left plus suspect portio. Abdominal hysterectomy with adnexae. A collum carcinoma was diagnosed histologically in the surgical preparation.

Case 64/9: The patient was operated on because of an 'uterine tumor'. In order to keep the intervention as small as possible, only supravaginal uterine amputation with removal of the right adnexa (the uterus is the size of a fist and already becomes detached on clamping). The patient died immediately after the intervention. At autopsy, an extensive collum carcinoma with hydroureter and hydronephrosis was diagnosed.

Emergency and Exploratory Laparotomies

In 33 terminal stages of collum carcinoma an anus praeter was applied. In 10 exploratory laparotomies, a collum carcinoma III was involved four times, an irradiated carcinoma three times, a relaparotomy after Wertheim operation once, a perforation in radium deposition once. Finally, the suspicion of an appendicitis in collum carcinoma III was not confirmed in 1 case. Two examples:

Case 97/1: Irradiated collum carcinoma III. Despite intensive radiotherapy, no effect on the tumor, therefore decision to operate. However, this proved to be impossible and only an exploratory laparotomy was carried out.

Case 212/9: Advanced collum carcinoma. After irradiation, decision to carry out laparotomy in order to remove the tumor at least partially. A uterus double the size of a fist and penetrated by carcinoma masses was found. Therefore limitation to exploratory laparotomy. The patient died as a result of pulmonary embolism soon after the operation.

Corpus Carcinoma

The 763 malignant tumors of the corpus uteri are the most numerous of the malignancies of the internal genitals which are operated on. Some women were first operated on with other diagnoses and the more grave affection was verified histologically after operation. This was a carcinoma in 703 cases, a sarcoma in 45, a carcinosarcoma in 13, and the simultaneous occurrence of a carcinoma and a sarcoma in 2 cases. The different morphological pictures have essentially the same clinical symptoms and for the sake of expediency are subsumed here under the term 'corpus carcinoma'.

The average age of the patients operated on was 67.5 years. 279 patients (36.6%) were aged from 60 to 64 years. 233 (30.5%) were 65–69 years old, 156 (20.5%) were 70–74 years old and 95 (12.4%) were at least 75 years old.

Abdominal or vaginal uterine extirpation with removal of the adnexae must be regarded as the only operation indicated here. Table 47 shows whether and how this demand could be met. The 477 abdominal hysterectomies with adnexae and the 148 vaginal hysterectomies with adnexae (in a further 60 vaginal hysterectomies the adnexae were left in) amount to 82.1% of all operations on corpus carcinoma. 6 Schauta operations, 4 Wertheim operations and 2 eviscerations are to be classified here, although one might dispute the usefulness of these interventions. The internal genitals were removed completely in 637 cases (83.5%). In the following are three examples of this.

Case 74/15: 'Because of postclimacterically occurring bleeding with a palpatory finding indicating a carcinoma corporis uteri, there is an indication for the Wertheim operation.' This intervention was performed without prior abrasion.

Case 76/15: 'Because of a corpus carcinoma verified by abrasion, a radical Wertheim hysterectomy was carried out. An infiltration into the parametria is not visible.'

Case 157/0: Portio PE: adenocarcinoma, Schauta operation without adnexae. Histology: corpus carcinoma.

Leaving the adnexae in place is sometimes expressively designated as 'exception' or 'contrary to the rule'. It is often not clear whether the vaginal access was correctly chosen preoperatively (e.g. 'because of the extraordinary difficulties of space, extirpation of the adnexae was dispensed with'). In our view it is not justifiable to 'leave the adnexae stumps in place to shorten the operation'. The ovaries are known often to be the first site of early metastasis of corpus carcinoma. Extirpation of the uterus leaving the adnexae in place must therefore be designated as wrong. It also cannot be justified by the shortening of the operation, which is in fact only insubstantial. In such a case, we would relaparotomize, remove the adnexae on both sides and work up the ovaries histologically.

Among the 29 palliative operations we classified 17 supravaginal uterine extirpations with or without adnexae, 10 'tumor extirpations' and 2 retrospective vaginal stump extirpations. They can be divided into two groups: (1) the interventions were not carried out by the surgeon to the planned extent for various (mostly technical) reasons, and (2) the operation was carried out with another preoperative diagnosis. We specify five cases as examples of this (609/0, 19/6, 64/6, 30/15).

Case 67/9: Despite the bleeding, a fractionated abrasion was refrained from and the patient laparotomized immediately under diagnosis of a uterus myomatosus: abdominal hysterectomy with adnexae. The justification of the demand to aim for a hysterectomy with adnexae after the menopause even in benign conditions, e.g. uterus myomatosus, is illustrated indirectly here.

The cases in which the operations were carried out under the assumption of a collum carcinoma constitute a special group.

Case 433/5: Because of an advanced portio carcinoma with infiltration of both parametria up to the pelvic wall (!), only a supravaginal uterine amputation without adnexae was possible. The histological examination then revealed a corpus carcinoma.

Case 406/2: Portio PE, adenocarcinoma of the cervix, vaginal hysterectomy with the adnexae proved to be a sufficient intervention only after histological diagnosis of a corpus carcinoma.

The 30 cases of exploratory laparotomy and 7 cases of emergency laparotomy do not need to be specially explained.

Tubal Carcinoma

Tubal carcinoma is not a typical geriatric malignancy. However, its rareness justifies clinical analysis of our 29 cases (table 48). The average age was 67.1 years. The oldest patient operated on was 73 years old.

4 patients without symptoms were recommended to undergo an operation at consultative examinations. 14 women complained of a bleeding of varying intensity and persistence. Only in 3 cases had this been designated expressly as smear bleeding or bloody discharge. We never found a note with regard to a hydrops tubae profluens. An abrasion was carried out 10 times. An adenocarcinoma was diagnosed 5 times, a sclerosed endometrium twice, an atrophic endometrium once and isolated epithelia were diagnosed once. No material could be obtained in an abrasion because of technical difficulties.

The preoperative diagnoses are noteworthy: ovarian carcinoma 5 times, hypogastric tumor 6 times, ovarian tumor twice, 'adnexal neoplasma' once, ovarian cyst 4 times, corpus carcinoma 3 times, adnexal tumor, uterus myomatosus, postmenopausal bleeding, total prolapse (tubal carcinoma as chance finding) once in each case. In 1 case, the preoperative diagnosis was not noted. Tubal carcinoma was assumed preoperatively only once and it was known from an earlier operation in only 2 cases.

The topical clinical problems of tubal carcinoma are best demonstrated by the surgical diagnoses: tubal carcinoma 10 times, ovarian carcinoma 4 times, ovarian tumor 3 times (tubal carcinoma once as a chance finding), adnexal tumor twice, corpus carcinoma twice, inoperable carcinoma, 'neoplasma', uterus myomatosus, pyosalpinx, sactosalpinx, ovarian tumor with hematosalpinx, 'posthorn-like distended tubes on both sides', 'blue transparent tubes the thickness of a thumb' once in each case.

Table 48. Tubal carcinoma in geriatric gynecological operation (in 169a)

No.	Case report No.	Age years	Symptoms	Abrasion	Preoperative diagnosis	Intraoperative diagnosis	Kind of operation	Histology No.	Exitus
1	52/0	62	full feeling for 4 weeks	−	ovarian cyst	ovarian carcinoma	abdominal hysterectomy with adnexae	962/60	−
2	307/0	63	hemorrhages for 14 days	adeno-carcinoma	'adenocarci-noma'	'tubes distended like posthorns on both sides'	Wertheim	1229/63	−
3	692/0	64	discharge tinged with blood for 4 weeks	adeno-carcinoma	neoplasm of adnexae	suspicion of neoplasm	abdominal hysterectomy with adnexae	1339/66	−
4	102/1	70	not traceable				salpingo-oopho-rectomy		later peritonitis
5	642/1	65	?		cystical ovarian tumor	ovarian carcinoma	abdominal hysterectomy with adnexae	23875/67	−
6	935/1	74	'becoming fat' over last 3 weeks		malignancy in lower abdomen	tubal carcinoma	exploratory laparotomy	27698/69	−
7	44/3	63	decrease in weight − abdominal pain		pancreatitis or tumor of lower abdomen	tubal carcinoma	salpingectomy	1933/60	
8	217/3	72	bleeding 2 years ago, now bleeding for last 2 weeks		postmenopausal bleeding with ovarian cystoma	tubal carcinoma and ovarian cyst	abdominal hysterectomy with adnexae	531/64	

9	436/3	66	bleeding for 8 days	sclerosed endometrium	ovarian tumor	ovarian tumor and hemosalpinx	abdominal hysterectomy with adnexae	3129/67
10	455/3	73	spotting for 6 months	sclerosed endometrium	tubal carcinoma	tubal carcinoma	abdominal hysterectomy with adnexae	331/67
11	429/3	62	total prolapse, increasing sinking symptoms, abrasion, perforation, laparotomy		total prolapse of cervical stump	total prolapse of cervical stump, and tubal carcinoma	stump extirpation with both adnexae	2298/67
12	334/4 373/4	64	abdominal hysterectomy with both adnexae 1 year ago		inoperable tubal carcinoma	inoperable tubal carcinoma	2 exploratory laparotomies	
13	414/4	63	consultative examination		tumor in lower abdomen	ovarian cystoma	salpingo-oophorectomy	262/68
14	509/5	67	consultative examination		tumor in lower abdomen	ovarian tumor	abdominal hysterectomy with adnexae	2340/68
15	10/6 45/6	60	bleeding for several months ambulant abrasion, adenocarcinoma	atrophic endometrium	corpus carcinoma	tumor of adnexae	supravaginal hysterectomy with adnexae, exploratory laparotomy	946/60
16	64/6	69	bleeding	–	tumor in lower abdomen	tubal carcinoma	supravaginal hysterectomy with adnexae	4997/61 –

Table 48 (continued)

No.	Case report No.	Age years	Symptoms	Abrasion	Preoperative diagnosis	Intraoperative diagnosis	Kind of operation	Histology No.	Exitus
17	116/6	61	bleeding abrasion	?	metrorrhagia in myomatous uterus	tubal carcinoma	exploratory laparotomy	2039/63	–
18	335/6	68	recurrent bleeding with 2 abrasions	adeno-carcinoma	corpus carcinoma	corpus carcinoma	vaginal hysterectomy with both adnexae	1614/68	–
19	379/6	69	vaginal hysterectomy 1 year ago with both adnexae (tubal carcinoma)		tubal carcinoma	inoperable carcinoma	exploratory laparotomy	60/69	cardio-vascular failure
20	83/7	68	consultative examination	–	ovarian carcinoma	ovarian cysts developed intraligamentally	abdominal hysterectomy with adnexae	33/69	–
21	112/7	71	increase in circumference of abdomen	–	ovarian carcinoma	inoperable carcinoma	exploratory laparotomy	34/65 only in autopsy	bronchial pneumonia
22	308/7	70	bleeding, increase in circumference of abdomen	adeno-carcinoma	ovarian carcinoma	ovarian carcinoma	salpingo-oophorectomy	2589/69	bronchial pneumonia
23	324/7	73	pressure in abdomen		ovarian carcinoma	adnexal tumor on both sides (pyosalpinx on both sides)	salpingo-oophorectomy on both sides	1039/69	–

24	234/9	65	consultative examination	–	ovarian tumor	myomatous uterus	abdominal hysterectomy with adnexae	2491/67	tumor cachexia
25	272/9	66	bleeding	adeno-carcinoma	corpus carcinoma	corpus carcinoma	abdominal hysterectomy with adnexae	2071/68	ileus
26	46/10	69	increase in circumference of abdomen, heavy bleeding	not technically possible	?	'blue transparent tubes the thickness of a thumb'	salpingectomy	996/61	–
27	338/14	65	bleeding	isolated epithelial splitters	postclimacteric bleeding	sactosalpinx the thickness of a finger	abdominal hysterectomy with adnexae	338/64	pulmonary embolism
28	69/14	69	spotting for 9 months	–	bleeding with tumor of adnexae	tubal carcinoma	abdominal hysterectomy with adnexae	1675/64	pulmonary embolism
29	49/15	69	supravaginal hysterectomy without adnexae because of myomatous uterus at age of 60; at 66, extirpation of vaginal stump because of adenocarcinoma of colon, now peritonitis	–	peritonitis in ovarian carcinoma	peritonitis in ovarian carcinoma	salpingo-oopho-rectomy	2780/61	peritonitis

In 14 cases, the internal genitals were completely removed abdominally. In the single vaginal hysterectomy carried out under the assumption of a corpus carcinoma, the importance of simultaneous removal of the adnexae is shown. The uterus with adnexae has been removed supravaginally in 2 cases. Otherwise, we noted 4 salpingo-oophorectomies, 2 salpingectomies and 7 exploratory laparotomies. In 8 fatalities (27.6%) there were the following causes of death: bronchopneumonia twice, pulmonary embolism twice, peritonitis, ileus, cardiovascular failures as well as tumor cachexia once in each case. We regard two cases as especially worthy of mention.

Case 26 (46/10): In the laparotomy the surgeon contented himself with a salpingectomy with a 'blue transparent tube the thickness of a thumb', although the abrasion which was aimed for because of a meat juice-colored discharge did not succeed for technical reasons, so that the course of the bleeding had to remain unelucidated.

Case 29 (49/15): In a 60-year-old patient both the cervix and the adnexae had to be left in place during the operation of a uterus myomatosus. 6 years later only the stump was removed because of a cervical carcinoma and the adnexae were left in place once again. 3 years later, the patient died in consequence of bronchopneumonia after operation on a perforated tubal carcinoma.

Ovarian Carcinoma

The 1,515 ovarian tumors are the second most frequent indication for surgery after genital displacements within this surgical material. The cases of extragenital conditions and uterus myomatosus also operated on after this diagnosis indicate the clinical importance of ovarian tumors.

The 604 ovarian malignancies (39.9% of all ovarian tumors) are the third most frequent gynecological malignancy operated on. In contrast to other malignant gynecological tumors, malignant ovarian tumors are of variable morphological structure. However, they are treated as a unit. The average age of the patients operated on was 67.9 years. Even here, the age alone does not decide on the kind of operation, so that an abdominal hysterectomy with complete removal of the adnexae is to be aimed for even in very old women.

Tables 42 and 47 give a survey of the surgical techniques. It is characteristic that abdominal hysterectomies with adnexae were carried out only 191 times (31.7%) and evisceration twice (0.3%).

We registered an incomplete intervention in the form of a palliative operation 236 times (39.1%). A supravaginal uterine amputation with complete or incomplete removal of the adnexae was involved 47 times and only an operation on the adnexae 189 times (51 tumor extirpations, 67 bilateral salpingo-oophorectomies and 71 unilateral salpingo-oophorectomies). Exploratory laparotomy is represented remarkably often with 156 cases (25.9%). The 19 emergency laparotomies (3.1%) round off the unsatisfactory picture on the surgical techniques in ovarian carcinomas.

On looking through all 604 surgical records, the so-called technical obstacles to hysterectomy with removal of the adnexae do not always appear convincing. We should like to underscore this view with some examples of relaparotomies in ovarian carcinomas:

Case 390/0: Ovarian carcinoma in 1962, adnexectomy on the right, recurrence in 1964. Relaparotomy, adnexectomy on the left (once again, no hysterectomy!).

Cases 118/1 and 220/1: Ovarian carcinoma 27.9.1961, adnexectomy on the left and myoma extirpation at the fundus. Recurrence 13.12.1962, relaparotomy, abdominal hysterectomy with remaining adnexae.

Case 416: Supravaginal uterine amputation with both adnexae in 1961, recurrence in 1964, stump extirpation.

Case 159/4: 'As already stated, the malignant tumor was well localized and could be extirpated in toto. Metastases 4 months later, abdominal hysterectomy with left tube.'

Case 89/5: At the age of 70, an appendectomy and cystectomy from the right ovary: 'After the appendectomy and freeing of adhesions, an ovarian cyst was emptied and several cysts of various size were visible. An extirpation of the entire cyst area was not carried out because of the condition of the patient.' Just a year later, there was a large lower abdominal abscess with ovarian carcinoma. Relaparotomy, drainage.

We also regard the following case histories as worthy of mention:

Case 82/10: Ovarian carcinoma on the left, adnexectomy on the left. 'The right adnexa and the uterus are unremarkable and therefore left in.'

Case 67/11: Metastasizing ovarian carcinoma with uterine descensus. Salpingo-oophorectomy on the right and antefixation of the uterus.

Case 130/1: Vaginal hysterectomy with right adnexa 2 years previously. Now ovarian carcinoma on the left.

Case 96/2: Abrasion 1 year previously, in which a 'myoma developed on the left' was suspected. Now an ovarian carcinoma the size of a human head on the left, ascites, adnexectomy on the left, ovarian adenocarcinoma, exitus 7 months later.

Timely laparotomy was very often neglected. This is proved among other things by the large number of exploratory laparotomies of which we have already treated the unsatisfactory results (196). In unclear palpation findings one should aim for diagnostic laparoscopy and be prepared to carry out laparotomy. The demand for intensification of the diagnostics for timely detection of ovarian tumors is thus to be made once more.

General Carcinoses

In this group we have included 37 patients in whom neither the site of operation nor the later histological examination could give adequate information on the primary localization of the malignancy. A few primary extragenital tumors are not to be excluded here, but the clinical problems are the same as those in advanced ovarian carcinomas. Tables 42 and 47 inform on individual kinds of operation. The origin of the malignant growth could not be clarified in 4 cases, even after abdominal hysterectomy with both adnexae.

Extragenital Intraperitoneal and Extraperitoneal Malignancies

The 125 extragenital malignancies (106 + 19) amount to 4.0% of all malignant tumors which were operated on. As expected, 68 cases of rectal and sigmoid carcinoma make up the majority. They have already been analyzed (198). At the head of the preoperative diagnoses are 'ovarian tumors' with 66 cases and 'hypogastric tumors' with 21 cases. Further preoperative diagnoses were: 5 adnexal tumors, 5 uterine tumors, 7 other tumors, and we did not find any concrete specification in 16 cases. Laparotomy was carried out by gynecologists five times under the diagnosis of a sigmoid carcinoma. We have already pointed out to the not yet fully exploited possibilities of preoperative diagnostics in co-operation with surgeons (192, 198).

Breast Cancer

With 1,125 cases, breast cancer is the most frequent carcinoma. After descensus vaginae et uteri, it is the most frequent condition which is operated on. Our material differs substantially in this point from previous data in the literature. A continuous rise in the number of breast operations can be observed over 10 years (1960: 69, 1969: 199). The proportion of breast operations in the surgical material of the individual hospital varied from 1.5% (department 11) to 32.6% (department 1). No breast operation was undertaken only in gynecology department 5.

On consideration of the 10-year period, it can be observed that the operation on breast cancer has been performed only sporadically in five small departments, but on the other hand to remarkably increasing extent in six large gynecology departments. For example, 374 operations (33.2% of all breast interventions) were performed in department 0. In department 1, 3 and 4 a further 429 breast cancer patients (38.1%) have been operated on. This means that 71.4% of all breast operations are to be registered in the four largest women's hospitals.

Noteworthy is the rising proportion of mammary carcinomas in relation to all illnesses from age group to age group: 60–64 years 30.1%, 65–69 years 33.0%, 70–74 years 39.0%, 75–79 years 43.7%, and 80 years and older 53.8%.

The duration of treatment of 47.7 days is determined by numerous factors in mammary carcinoma. We thus found quite different data within individual clinics (varying between 20.2 and 55.9 days). Some small clinics are not representative because of few cases and the lack of possibility of postoperative treatment. The duration of preoperative treatment (3.6–10.5 days) was possibly influenced slightly in a few clinics by the irradiation which was brought forward in the early years of the period evaluated. Large differences are found in the departments in the postoperative period (16.6–48.7 days), since in some cases there was no possibility of irradiation, the kind or number of the irradiation varied, the irradiation was only commenced in hospitalized patients or had been terminated, etc. In the individual years, we find a tendency to reduction in the average duration of postoperative treatment. This is shown in particular by the division into two groups of the cases in surgical material which did not die and depending on the time of operation: in 1960–1964, an average duration of treatment of 52.5 days (7.6 + 44.9) was found in 423 cases, and in 1965–1969, there was an average duration of 44.2 days (8.0 + 36.2) in 674 cases.

Age alone does not constitute a contraindication to surgical treatment of breast cancer. Thus hormone treatment and application of cytostatics can only constitute an additional method of treatment, even in elderly women.

By comparing our material with the literature on surgical geriatric gynecology, we have found only 14 communications with data on 277 breast operations. These are not representative for the geriatric significance of the malignancy, since they are in part papers from a time in which the gynecologist was hardly involved in the surgical treatment of breast cancer, and breast operations are often not included in the surgical material analyzed.

Our material shows that the surgical treatment of breast cancer has in the meantime become a routine operation in large gynecology departments. However, it is not necessary that this operation should also spread into the small gynecology departments, which do not have direct facilities for making rapid histological sections or for postoperative irradiation.

Benign Tumors

The 1,141 benign tumors operated on constitute 17.1% of the entire material. By far the most frequent benign tumors were the ovarian tumors (911 cases) and uterus myomatosus (193 cases) (table 49). The 20 benign vulvar tumors and 1 vaginal cyst which were operated on are not representative. The interventions have mostly been designated as 'small', and we have not recorded the absolute number. The 7 benign extragenital intraperitoneally located tumors involved 3 myomas and 1 neurinoma of the small intestine, a 'spleen tumor' in a retrospectively diagnosed leukemia, an omentum lipoma and a xanthofibroma peritonei. The 9 benign extraperitoneal processes exclusively concerned retroperitoneally situated organs.

Uterus myomatosus

In 193 cases a uterus myomatosus diagnosed before or during the operation was the only indication or the main indication for surgery (table 50). Only 89 women (47.0%) were operated on after the diagnosis 'uterus myomatosus'. In 31 cases (16.4%) the preoperative diagnosis was 'tumor of the lower abdomen' or 'ovarian tumor' or 'uterus myomatosus'. In 60 women (31.8%) the operation was performed under the assumption of an ovarian tumor.

Table 49. Age groups, average age and duration of treatment in various diseases

Diseases	Total cases	Age groups, years										Average age, years	Average duration of treatment, days		
		60–64		65–69		70–74		75–79		80 and over			total	before operation	after operation
		n	%	n	%	n	%	n	%	n	%				
Uterus myomatosus	193	66	34.2	63	32.6	43	22.3	19	9.8	2	1.0	67.4	38.0	9.1	28.9
Benign ovarian tumors	911	307	33.7	260	28.5	218	23.9	93	10.2	33	3.6	68.0	34.4	8.8	25.6
Inflammatory diseases	40	23	57.5	12	30.0	2	5.0	3	7.5	–	–	65.2	40.9	12.0	28.9
Carcinoma *in situ*	65	37	56.9	18	27.7	6	9.2	3	4.6	1	1.5	64.8	39.6	13.7	25.9
Uterine bleeding	44	20	45.5	10	22.7	7	15.9	6	13.6	1	2.3	67.0	34.9	9.1	25.8
Urogenital fistulae	42	22	52.4	9	21.4	8	19.0	3	7.1	–	–	65.8	41.3	3.0	38.3
Appendicitis	48	28	58.3	10	20.8	3	6.3	4	8.3	3	6.3	65.8	29.6	7.8	21.8
Sigmoid diverticulitis	49	17	34.7	15	20.8	9	18.4	7	14.3	1	2.0	67.7	38.2	10.0	28.2

Table 50. Operations in uterus myomatosus

Crucial kind of operation	Cases		Removal of adnexae present		Postoperative mortality	
	n	%	complete	incomplete or none	cases	%
Vaginal hysterectomy	11	5.7	0	11	–	–
Abdominal hysterectomy	124	64.3	107	17	5	4.0
Supravaginal uterine amputation	41	21.2	20	21	3	7.3
Abdominal stump extirpation	1	0.5	1	0	–	–
Myoma enucleation	16	8.3	0	16	–	–
Total	193	100.0	128	65	8	4.1

The diagnosis uterus myomatosus was made in more than half the cases on the basis of an isolated node. Surgical preparations with several nodes are frequently described, one node always being larger than the others. In detailed surgical reports, the isolated nodes have often been described as intraligamentally developed myomas (20 cases).

Apart from a few exceptions, in which a calcified subserous myoma node 'the size of a pullet egg' was the indication for laparotomy, myomas can often be quite large. The surgeons or pathologists describe uterus myomatosus as 'the size of a man's fist' in 32 cases, 'the size of 2 fists' in 16 cases, 'the size of a child's head' in 21 cases, 'the size of a man's head' in 9 cases, and 'the size of a coconut' in 6 cases. The uterus reached as far as the navel five times and was 'the size of a handball' in 4 cases (573/01, 734/01, 838/01, 979/01). In other cases, the size of the uterus is stated to be 20 × 16 × 10 cm (105/00), 20 × 17 × 14 cm (300/00), 20 × 14 × 10 cm (438/00), 30 × 25 cm (223/05), and the weight was stated to be 1,920 g (162/03), 2,000 g (496/05), 2,100 g (43/15) up to 7,000 g (355/00).

Hysterectomy was carried out a total of 135 times (70.0%) (vaginally 11 times and abdominally 124 times). The adnexae were removed at the same time in only 107 cases. The view of *Benthin* (400) that supravaginal uterine amputation in myomas after menopause is not only the most gentle but also the most readily overseen has mere historical importance. This also applies in geriatric patients with a uterus myomatosus. Nevertheless, we still found 41 cases (21.2%) of supravaginal uterine amputations. In 16 cases (8.3%) the intervention was limited to removal of a myoma node. A connection between the frequency of individual surgical techniques and the age of the patients is not discernible.

The evaluation of our cases contradicts the hypothesis of the postmenopausal involution of the larger myomas. Accordingly, extirpation of a uterus myomatosus cannot be regarded as a typically geriatric gynecologic operation, since the intervention should have been undertaken in many cases at a much earlier time, or in some cases it could have been avoided when all the possibilities of diagnosis had been employed.

The operation was only recommended on the occasion of a cancer prevention or consultative examination in a remarkably large number of the 193 patients. This indicates that a large proportion of the women had probably not visited a gynecologist for a long time.

In our opinion, 21.2% supravaginal uterine amputations in uterus myomatosus is too high, even in elderly women. To our surprise, the adnexae were only removed along with the uterus in 128 cases (66.3%). They were left in place not because of the severity of the intervention or to shorten the operation, but because they were 'normal', 'intact', 'senile', 'in order' etc. We found a corresponding note only at *Knörr et al.* (3) with the recommendation that the adnexae should be removed along with the uterus as prophylaxis against carcinoma in the postmenopause in myoma patients.

Benign Ovarian Tumors

Benign ovarian tumors were by far the most frequent benign growth (911 cases) in our operation material. Table 51 gives a general survey of the methods of operation in benign ovarian tumors. The kind of operation was mostly clinic-linked and only partly dependent on age.

We found abdominal hysterectomy with removal of the adnexae in 328 cases and other operations with complete removal of the remaining internal genitals in 21 cases. Bilateral salpingo-oophorectomies (109 cases) can only be regarded as an adequate operation in pronounced multimorbidity or very old women. In such cases, a fractionated abrasion must be carried out previously without fail. We have often failed to find this meticulousness in the present material.

We consider that the procedure was unjustified in 54 cases in which an adnexa operation was combined with a supravaginal uterine amputation. In a benign ovarian tumor, preparing out and extirpating the mostly atrophic cervic should not constitute a technical problem. We have objections in principle against the 403 unilateral oophorectomies (44.7%). It can be suspected that an ovarian tumor is benign on the basis of its macroscopic constitution, but this can be verified only by histological examination. The surgeon must be aware in each individual case of the whole problem of primary and secondary multiplicity with cancerization of ovarian tumors.

Table 51. Operations in benign ovarian tumors

Crucial kind of operation	Cases		Removal of adnexae present		Postoperative mortality	
	n	%	complete	incomplete or none	n	%
Abdominal hysterectomy	328	36.4	327	1	14	4.3
Abdominal stump extirpation	7	0.8	7	0	1	14.3
Supravaginal uterine amputation	54	6.0	42	12	6	11.1
Bilateral salpingo-oophorectomy	109	12.1	109[1]	0	3	2.8
Unilateral salpingo-oophorectomy	403	44.7	32[2]	371	22	5.5
Total	901[3]	100.0	517	384	46	5.1

[1] No uterus present in 10 cases.
[2] No uterus present in 4 cases.
[3] 10 cases of vaginal operation not taken into account.

We mention as examples of primary methods of examination which are not consistently chosen:

Case 1026/0: Cystadenoma of the right ovary, adnexectomy on the right. Abrasion carried out after recurrent smear bleeding for almost a year: carcinoma corporis uteri.

Case 268/2: Bleeding in the postmenopause. 'Suspicion of a corpus tumor.' An ovarian tumor was diagnosed under inpatient observation. No abrasion, but what unilateral adnexectomy was performed: multilocular ovarian cystoma.

Case 34/10: Ovarian cyst on the left, uterus is missing, ovarectomy on the left and appendectomy. Right adnexa left in place, 'the appendix appears to be unchanged in external appearance, but is removed in the usual way'.

Case 90/11: Total prolapse of the uterus, ovarian tumor on the right. Therefore only salpingo-oophorectomy and corpus fixation. 'The left adnexae are healthy (only several quite small cysts up to the size of beans are found).'

Case 334/5: In 1957, clinical suspicion of an ovarian carcinoma. Exploratory laparotomy, fibroma demonstrated histologically, 40 precautionary 'irradiations'. In 1975, cystadenoma of the ovary on both sides. Relaparotomy, supravaginal uterine amputation with both adnexae.

Case 249/8: Cystoma of the ovary on the left, adnexectomy on the left plus appendectomy.

Case 135/10: Ovarian cystoma: 'Tumor was amputated from the ovary: appendectomy.'

Non-Palpable and Hormonally Active Ovarian Tumors

Because of the specific geriatric problems, the non-palpable and hormonally active ovarian tumors will be discussed here. First of all, small but palpable tumors must be distinguished from the non-palpable tumors in macroscopically normal ovaries. We refer to the paper by *Erb* (337) for the diagnostic and therapeutic procedure in small ovarian tumors.

The non-palpable ovarian tumors are occasionally hormonally active and then become noticeable by bleeding in the postmenopause or in the senium (324, 332, 354). *Behrens* (325) observed 9 genital bleedings in consequence of very small hormonally active ovarian tumors in the course of 10 years at the Leipzig University Gynecology Department. These tumors could not be diagnosed by palpation. *Kyank* (365) described an especially small granulosa cell tumor as the cause of a recurrent glandular hyperplasia after radiological castration.

An impressive case of a small androgenically active ovarian tumor was published by *Groot-Wassink et al.* (349). With typical symptoms, there was at first a normal gynecological palpation finding, and laparoscopy also revealed macroscopically unsuspicious ovaries. The final demonstration of the ovarian tumor only succeeded after catheterization of the femoral vein and selective withdrawals of venous blood through determinations of testosterone in the plasma of the individual fractions. Microscopically, *Dhom* (335) as well as *Jalůvka and Kratzsch* (358) among others found small Brenner tumors. *Vácha and Kopečný* (393) describe 7 cases of carcinomas in macroscopically unaltered ovaries. The authors recommend that 'normal ovaries' should also be removed when there is peritoneal carcinosis without unequivocal localization of the primary tumor.

In our material, 56 ovarian tumors have been designated as hormonally active on the basis of the histological examination. These were 32 granulosa cell tumors, 10 granulosa cell carcinoms, 8 theca cell tumors, and 6 Löffler-Priesel tumors. The results of a fresh examination of the patient records of appropriate patients will be published later *(Felshart and Jalůvka)*. Therefore only some data on the anamneses and preoperative diagnostics are given here.

A cytological vaginal smear was never instituted preoperatively. We also noted the lack of any preoperative hormonal examination in all cases. Out of the 56 patients, 35 (62.5%) reported no bleeding and 21 (37.5%) a single bleeding before admission.

In the 36 hormonally active ovarian tumors without bleeding, 35 women were admitted and operated with the diagnosis of an ovarian tumor. An exception is assumed appendicitis. Abdominal hysterectomy with both adnexae was performed 21 times. Otherwise, 3 supravaginal uterine amputations with adnexectomy, 10 salpingo-oophorectomies or tumor extirpations and 1 exploratory laparotomy were performed; in 1 case, an anus praeter was applied.

In the 11 patients with bleeding without abrasion before laparotomy, the referral diagnoses were diverse: metrorrhagia 6 times, uterus myomatosus once, suspicion of function tumor twice, an acute abdomen and a suspect portio once in each case. Clinical diagnosis before the intervention: ovarian tumors 5 times, function tumors twice and uterus myomatosus 4 times. Despite the presence of bleeding and the fact that abrasion was not performed, the surgeons contented themselves 3 times with tumor extirpation (a possible corpus carcinoma could not be eliminated in this way) and once with a supravaginal uterine amputation and adnexectomy.

In 10 women with metrorrhagias an abrasion was carried out before the operation. The referral diagnoses were: bleedings 5 times, ovarian tumors 4 times and uterus myomatosus once. The histological examinations revealed: 5 glandular cystic hyperplasias, 3 corpus carcinomas, 1 corpus carcinoma polyp without description of the endometrium, and 1 'matron's polyp, no hormone stimulation'. The indications for surgery were: 4 ovarian tumors, 2 function tumors, 3 corpus carcinomas and 1 uterus myomatosus. We noted 7 abdominal hysterectomies with adnexae, 2 supravaginal uterine amputations with adnexae (corpus carcinoma polyp, uterus myomatosus), and 1 unilateral adnexectomy (matron's polyps). The 90-year-old patient (12/17) is as far as we know the oldest patient with a granulosa cell carcinoma to have been operated on (356).

In the literature, many authors assume a hormonal activity of some Brenner tumors (358). In our material, 17 Brenner tumors have been verified histologically. 2 patients reported a metrorrhagia before admission. In case 267/6, abrasion revealed a corpus polyp. There followed supravaginal uterine amputation with both adnexae. In case 317/6, only bilateral oophorectomy was carried out despite the bleeding.

The hormonal activity of the Brenner tumors has in our opinion not yet been adequately proved. It has mostly been assumed only on the basis of the postmenopausal bleeding or bleeding in the senium. Some authors find shifts in the endocrine cytological smears. The demonstration of Sudan-positive lipid substances may also indicate the hormonal activity of some Brenner tumors. Hormone determination has so far been carried out rarely and only before the operation. In this connection one should not forget the activity of the adrenal cortex which is typical for advanced age. We operated on a Brenner tumor with recurrent glandular-cystic hyperplasias (two abrasions) and pathological estrogen excretion in a patient with advanced mammary carcinoma. The estrogen excretions still remain greatly elevated 2 years after abdominal hysterectomy with adnexae. On autopsy, a metastasis of the breast cancer in one adrenal cortex was found (358). Further studies are necessary to clarify the question of facultative hormonal activity of Brenner tumors.

At every bleeding in the menopause and in the senium, a fractionated abrasion is absolutely necessary. In a corresponding histological finding, one must also think of a hormonally active ovarian tumor even with an otherwise normal palpation finding and one must aim for complete extirpation of the internal genitals. Preoperative hormone determination is greatly recommended. In the literature, data are lacking on the relations between endometrium state and estrogen excretion in women who are no longer menstruating. It would be worthwhile for clinics with histological and endocrinological laboratories or departments to fill this gap.

Ovarian tumors have sometimes only been diagnosed as hormonally active on the basis of the histological examination of the surgical preparation. Comparison of preoperative and postoperative hormone excretion is then no longer possible. Specific hormone examinations have been rarely undertaken routinely in all ovarian tumors (323, 326–328, 336, 343, 353, 360, 361, 368, 372, 380, 383, 392, 398, 399). Further clinical endocrinological information is also to be expected here.

Other Gynecological Diseases

The small absolute number of the 266 clinical pictures to be classified here only enables a global analysis (table 49). After registering the material from the years 1970 to 1979, we hope to be able to analyze this geriatric gynecological pathology separately.

In 40 inflammatory processes in the region of the internal genitals, a pyometra was involved 6 times. Under the collective term 'inflammatory adnexal diseases', we find 34 conglomerate tumors, adhesions in the adnexal area, pyosalpinges and tuboovarian abscesses. In the majority of the cases, the women were laparotomized under other diagnoses (mostly ovarian tumor). This is also reflected in the operations performed: exclusively adhesiolyses 9 times, exploratory laparotomies 4 times (perhaps also with adhesiolyses, exitus 3 times), abdominal hysterectomies with adnexae 10 times and adnexectomies 10 times. We pointed out the dangers of adhesiolysis in inflammatory conditions in an earlier publication (198). The new possibilities of diagnosis, e.g. laparoscopy, make this group of diseases worthy of clinical attention.

We recorded 65 hysterectomies in patients with carcinoma in situ or a surface carcinoma of the portio. 53 operations were performed in three women's hospitals and 12 operations in eight women's hospitals. In seven hospitals, this precancerous condition in elderly women was evidently not regarded as a sufficient indication for uterine extirpation. The small number of carcinomas in situ in our operation material can only be partially explained by this fact. We assume in agreement with *Wittlinger* (318) that precancerous conditions only rarely arise in elderly women. In 65 hysterectomies, the adnexae were removed at the same time only 37 times (56.9%). As in other clinical pictures, the dissimilar procedure in abdominally and vaginally operated patients is notice-able. In 31 abdominal hysterectomies, the adnexae were left in place twice, and in 34 vaginal hysterectomies the adnexae were left in place in 26 cases because of the same precancerous condition.

In a few cases, a carcinoma in situ was diagnosed by chance or retrospective-ly without previous conization:

Case 222/12: Descensus vaginae et uteri. Portio erosion. Manchester operation and colporrhaphies. Histology: carcinoma in situ.

Case 2987/7: Suspect portio with PAP IV. Immediate vaginal hysterectomy with adnexae. Histology. carcinoma in situ.

Case 79/11: Pressure ulcer in prolapsus vaginae et portionis. Exploratory excision. Carcinoma in situ. Three radium implantations with 4,000 mgeh, afterwards fixation of the abdominal stump to the rectus abdominis muscles and salpingo-oophorectomy on the left. Adhesiolysis.

Case 123/2: Suspect portio, vaginal hysterectomy without adnexae. 'Because of a suspect portio resulting from several cytological smears, we carried out a vaginal hyster-ectomy. The histology revealed a superficial carcinoma of the portio. The surgical interven-tion can thus be regarded as optimal.' The procedure would have been insufficient in invasive carcinoma.

A recurrent bleeding was the main indication for hysterectomy 44 times. The intervention was performed either primarily or with benign histology. It is questionable that the adnexae were only removed at the same time 22 times, 17 times in 20 abdominal hysterectomies and only 3 times in 24 vaginal hyster-ectomies. In the same disease, a uniform attitude concerning the extent of the intervention should prevail. This applies all the more when one has to think of the possibility of a non-palpable hormonally active ovarian tumor. Precisely in this group (assuming technical difficulties in vaginal adnexectomy) laparotomy should be given preference and one should not dispense with salpingo-oophorectomy.

We should like to mention only one case (126/14) among 15 operated uterine perforations. External abrasion: 'Bleeding not brought to a stop. For this reason, I regard a radium implantation as urgently indicated.' Correct diagnosis: uterine perforation; vaginal hysterectomy without adnexae.

The 15 cases of kraurosis or leukoplakia of the vulva, 13 cases of suspect portio and 65 cases of carcinoma in situ which we registered cannot convey the correct picture concerning the quantitative occurrence of these precancerous conditions in geriatric gynecological patients. For this purpose, the complete registration of the small interventions would have been necessary. In the other 25 different gynecological conditions, normal internal genitals were shown intraoperatively 11 times, although a pathological finding (mostly an ovarian tumor) was suspected preoperatively. Very rare clinical pictures were involved 14 times.

Other Surgical Diseases

Here we content ourselves with a synopsis (table 49) of the evaluation of 147 surgical diseases already presented (192).

Extragenital Diseases

From a gynecological point of view, a classification of the operations on extragenital diseases into three groups suggested itself: conditions primarily operated on by gynecologists; disease diagnosed during a laparotomy, and diseases operated on additionally in gynecological interventions. With an all-embracing interpretation of the term 'extragenital diseases in surgical gynecology', yet another group would have to be taken into account, i.e. extragenital interventions which are necessary in gynecological diseases.

Our patients include 282 women with an extragenital disease (4.2%) who were operated on mainly under gynecological diagnoses. We have already dealt with the problems of these cases in an earlier publication (192). In extragenital diseases, a subdivision into intraperitoneal and extraperitoneal (or retroperitoneal) clinical pictures is to be recommended. Especially the latter pathological findings often cause the gynecologist great difficulties in differential diagnosis because of their rareness.

We suggest that the retroperitoneal diseases as seen by the gynecologist should be divided into six groups (193):

1   Malignant and benign primary retroperitoneal tumors
2   Retroperitoneally situated organs
3   Malignant and benign tumors of retroperitoneally situated organs
4   Retroperitoneal gynecological structures
5   Retroperitoneal metastases
6   Other diseases in the retroperitoneal space

We are also able to confirm the clinical applicability of this classification in our geriatric surgical patients (193). We refer to our already cited papers regarding the relatively sporadic reports in the geriatric gynecological literature on operations on extragenital intraperitoneal and retroperitoneal diseases.

Additionally Operated Diseases

We agree with *Wittlinger* (318) that the multiple morbidity which is so typical, e.g. in internal medicine, is not very pronounced in gynecology. Nevertheless, we were able to list 266 cases (4.0%) (table 52) where besides a

Table 52. Diseases operated on in addition

Diseases	Total cases	Main indication				
		genital dis- place- ments	malig- nant tumors	benign tumors	other gyneco- logical diseases	other surgical diseases
Genital displacements	40	–	14	26	–	–
Malignant gynecological tumors	24	6	12	3	2	1
Malignant surgical tumors	7	1	3	3	–	–
Benign gynecological tumors	89	20	30	34	2	3
Benign surgical tumors	2	–	–	2	–	–
Other gynecological diseases	8	2	1	3	–	2
Other surgical diseases	96	16	29	43	5	3
None						
cases	6,393	1,948	3,024	1,027	256	138
%	96.0	97.7	97.1	90.0	96.6	93.9
Total cases	6,659	1,993	3,113	1,141	265	147

gynecological condition, other gynecological or surgical conditions were operated on.

Three additional diseases operated on at the same time were the most frequent: benign gynecological tumors (mostly ovarian tumors), genital displacements, and assumed appendicitis. We have not recorded the numerous cases of uterus myomatosus as an additional disease, e.g. in a corpus carcinoma; this will be done in the second analysis. The group of malignancies additionally operated on was quantitatively small, but very much more illuminating. This group included 24 gynecological and 7 surgical malignant tumors. Geriatric gynecological patients afford especially good conditions for systematic examination of collision tumors and combination tumors.

In complete operations, e.g. a hysterectomy with adnexae or even with colporrhaphy operations, the basic gynecological conditions can be treated causally, and also the additional gynecological disease at the same time. This contrasts with other disciplines, especially internal medicine. There is no objection in principle to surgical treatment of an additional surgical condition. The precondition for this is complete surgical clearing of the genital organs, i.e. treatment of the basic disease. This requirement is only rarely met.

Postoperative Mortality

Of 6,658 patients operated on, 511 women (7.7%) died postoperatively. The high postoperative mortality compared to the literature does not justify negative conclusions with regard to the care of patients in West Berlin gynecology departments. We have refrained from any statistical rectification of the postoperative mortality (see the General Chapter). The 493 patient records which are not available indicate that patients either received outpatient post-operative follow-up treatment or had been hospitalized once more. The post-operative mortality in all 7,151 patients operated on would thus be somewhat lower (7.1–7.7%).

In individual years, the mortality varied between 5.1 and 11.2%. The lowest rates were recorded in 1968 (5.7%) and 1969 (5.1%). The differences are not significant. By forming two 5-year groups (1960–1964 and 1965–1969) we determined a postoperative mortality of 8.4 and 7.2%, respectively. However, it is not certain that a decline in the postoperative mortality was involved; the alterations in the surgical patients may play an appreciable role. An example for this is the increase in breast cancer operations, which have a low postoperative mortality.

The postoperative mortality varied between 1.1 and 16.3% in the individual gynecology departments. These extreme values are due to the small absolute figures. A significant difference between the mortality rates of the gynecology departments does not exist.

We detected a slight dependence of the postoperative mortality on age: in 60- to 64-year-old patients the mortality was 5.9%, in 65- to 69-year-old patients 7.8%, in 70- to 74-year-old patients 8.7%, in 75- to 79-year-old patients 8.9%, and in 80-year-old and older patients 13.8%. The attempt was doubtless made to choose simple methods of operation in the presence of multiple morbidity. However, detailed analyses revealed that the postoperative mortality is no longer dependent on the extent and thus the duration of the intervention. 395 patients (77.3%) died in the first 28 postoperative days and 116 (22.7%) died later. If the latter deaths are not taken into account, our postoperative mortality would be only 5.9 instead of 7.7%. Up to the 7th postoperative day, 204 women (39.9%) died, between the 8th and 14th postoperative day there were 113 (22.1%), between the 15th and 21st postoperative day 47 (9.2%), and between the 22nd and the 28th postoperative day 31 women died (6.1%).

Frequency of Autopsy

Out of 511 women who died, 282 (55.2%) were autopsied. An autopsy was dispensed with 135 times (26.4%), it was refused 25 times (4.9%) and we have not found any autopsy data 69 times (13.5%). The 229 women who were not autopsied amount to 44.8% of all patients who died postoperatively. In our opinion, this percentage is too high. Precisely in elderly patients, the complication leading to death should always be accurately determined. Only in this way can it be decided whether the death was primarily due to the basic disease or whether it had been caused by an unexpected complication or by an insufficient preoperative preparation, an intervention which had not been chosen optimally or by inconsistent treatment of postoperative complications.

We found the lowest autopsy rate in 1968 (41.3%) and the highest in 1966 (66.7%). The differences cannot be interpreted unequivocally. This also applies to the two 5-year groups: 1960–1964 (53.5% autopsies) and 1965–1969 (56.5% autopsies). The frequency of autopsy falls continuously with increasing time between the operation and exitus. We recorded a decline in autopsy rate with increase in age of patients: of women who died between 60 and 64 years of age, the autopsy rate was 55.2%, in 65- to 69-year-old women it was 59.9%, in 70- to 74-year-old women 53.8%, in 75- to 79-year-old women 51.7% and in 80-year-old and older women the autopsy rate was 44.4%. The great age of the operated women who died should not affect the decision to carry out an autopsy.

We found significant differences in the autopsy rate in the individual hospitals. In the three gynecology departments, autopsy was carried out in no case among 22 deaths and was carried out 8 times in four gynecology departments with 86 deaths. These 108 deaths with 8 autopsies (7.4%) from seven gynecology departments contrast with 403 deaths with 274 autopsies (68.0%) from ten gynecology departments. In our opinion, the complication leading to exitus should be explained in terms of pathological anatomy even when the primary disease is known. Less restraint in the autopsy patients who have died after geriatric gynecological operations would be desirable.

Individual Causes of Death

In designing table 53 we took into account both the data in the literature and the causes of death specified in the case records.

Cardiovascular Failure. This was the most frequent cause of death with 103 cases (20.2%). We have already expressed our reservations with regard to the reliability of this concept as a cause of death (190), as well as mentioning it in the General Chapter of this article. Analysis of our material has completely confirmed these misgivings. 93 of these women (90.3%) were not autopsied! They constitue 40.6% of all non-autopsied patients who died postoperatively. Conversely, the 10 autopsy cases (9.7%) make up only 3.5% of all autopsied women. One might also specify other causes here. For example, of 9 patients

Table 53. Autopsy frequency in individual causes of death

Cause of death	All fatalities			Autopsy				
	cases	%		yes			no	
		1	2	cases	%		cases	%
					1	2	1	2
'Cardiovascular failure'	103	100	20.2	10	9.7	3.5	93	90.3	40.6
Pulmonary embolism	90	100	17.6	68	75.6	24.1	22	24.4	9.6
Tumor cachexia	75	100	14.7	38	50.7	13.5	37	49.3	16.2
Peritonitis	72	100	14.1	60	83.3	21.3	12	16.7	5.2
Bronchopneumonia	44	100	8.6	30	68.2	10.6	14	31.8	6.1
Organic diseases of cardiovascular system	35	100	6.8	21	60.0	7.4	14	40.0	6.1
Ileus	35	100	6.8	16	45.7	5.7	19	54.3	8.3
'Immediate mortality'	25	100	4.9	16	64.0	5.7	9	36.0	4.0
Kidney failure	18	100	3.5	13	72.2	4.7	5	27.8	2.2
Other causes	14	100	2.7	10	71.4	3.5	4	28.6	1.7
Total	511	100	100.0	282	55.2	100.0	229	44.8	100.0

with malignancies, 3 died of postoperative shock immediately after an exploratory laparotomy. The cause of death 124 days after an exploratory laparotomy in inoperable kidney carcinoma should actually have been specified as tumor cachexia. We should like to repeat emphatically our view that cardiovascular failure is practically always only the immediate cause of death and not the postoperative complication leading to exitus.

Pulmonary Embolism. From a total of 90 cases (17.6%), this was verified 68 times (75.6%) by autopsy. In 23.8% of all autopsied women, a pulmonary embolism was the cause of death. In view of its characteristic symptoms, it can be assumed that the clinical diagnosis is correct even in the majority of the 22 women not autopsied.

Tumor Cachexia. With 75 cases (14.7%) this takes third place. 37 women (49.3%) were not autopsied. In our opinion, if tumor cachexia were consistently taken into account, it would make up a considerable proportion of the postoperative mortality. Because cachexia can only occur in malignancies, it is relatively infrequently represented in the total statistics. If the proportion of tumor cachexia is too high, one might have certain misgivings with regard to the indication for surgical treatment of advanced malignancies.

Peritonitis. The 72 women who died of peritonitis after laparotomy make up 14.1% of the total postoperative mortality. We listed the highest proportion (83.3%) of autopsies here.

Bronchopneumonia. Of 44 cases of lethal bronchopneumonia (8.6%), 30 (68.2%) have been verified by autopsy. The greater predisposition of old women for postoperative bronchopneumonia has certainly played a role here.

Organic Cardiovascular Diseases. The 35 cases (6.8%) do not constitute a homogeneous cause of death. They result either from a disease which was already present before the operation or from a cardiovascular complication which has only arisen after the operation: 7 cardiac insufficiencies, 2 arrhythmias, 7 myocardial infarctions (no autopsy 3 times), 1 pulmonary edema, 3 arterial sclerosis and 1 hypertension. A cerebral hemorrhage or thrombosis was diagnosed 14 times.

Ileus. Out of 35 women who died with ileus symptoms, only 16 (45.7%) were autopsied. The importance of this grave postoperative complication is treated on page 141.

Immediate Mortality. This term used as specified in the literature has not proved to be appropriate. The 25 deaths (4.9%) proved to be mostly postoperative shock and only rarely a real anesthetic incident.

We have already pointed out the possibilities of postoperative care in our material which are still available with the analysis of the early mortality: 86 women (16.8% of all deaths or 1.3% of all patients operated on) died on the day of the operation or during the first 3 days afterwards, i.e. they are to be evaluated as cases of early mortality (199). Especially in unexpected deaths which have occurred immediately after the operation, the question arises epicritically as to the indication for surgery. The interventions were always indicated in our patients. A part from a few collum carcinoma operations, there are no objections to the procedures chosen. In consideration of the prior injuries, the preoperative state and the preparation, two factors were noticeable: (1) the frequent pathological changes in the vessels, the heart and the lungs, and (2) the rare application of preoperative measures for improvement of cardiac activity and pulmonary function (digitalis, respiration therapy by means of physical measures and drugs).

After analysis of our material, we can accept without reservations the views of *Schulze* (275) and *Kviz* (211) concerning the minor role of anesthesia in intraoperative and postoperative mortality in gynecological interventions. From the available documentation we were occasionally able to observe an unusual performance of the anesthesia, but there was a definite link between the exitus

Table 54. Duration of postoperative treatment in individual causes of death

Cause of death	Total cases	Duration of postoperative treatment, days										Average duration days	Median value days
		0–7		8–14		15–21		22–28		29 and over			
		n	%	n	%	n	%	n	%	n	%		
'Immediate mortality'	25	25	100.0	–	–	–	–	–	–	–	–	0.6	0.0
'Cardiovascular failure'	103	40	38.8	26	25.2	10	9.7	8	7.8	19	18.4	16.2	8.8
Organic diseases of cardiovascular system	35	9	25.7	6	17.1	1	2.9	5	14.3	14	40.0	28.0	23.9
Pulmonary embolism	90	32	35.6	24	26.7	15	16.7	4	4.4	15	16.7	17.1	10.8
Bronchopneumonia	44	19	43.2	14	31.8	3	6.8	–	–	8	18.2	18.7	8.3
Kidney failure	18	6	33.3	3	16.7	3	16.7	2	11.1	4	22.2	23.9	15.5
Peritonitis	72	39	54.2	17	23.6	9	12.5	2	2.8	5	6.9	10.7	7.1
Ileus	35	22	62.9	10	28.6	1	2.9	1	2.9	1	2.9	8.6	6.6
Tumor cachexia	75	8	10.7	9	12.0	3	4.0	9	12.0	46	61.3	49.1	44.6
Other causes	14	4	28.6	4	28.6	2	14.3	–	–	4	28.6	21.1	13.0
Total	511	204	39.9	113	22.1	47	9.2	31	6.1	116	22.7	–	–

and the anesthesia in only one case. This knowledge is important, since the anesthesia in our operation material could not yet be given by anesthetists, and the gynecological surgeon often had to bear responsibility for the anesthesia. Even in the 6 cases of intraoperative death we were unable to detect an immediate effect of the anesthesia as the sole cause of the lethal outcome.

Kidney Failure. In 18 cases of lethal kidney failure (3.5%) the terminal stage of a malignancy was involved 13 times and the terminal stage of a kidney disease 5 times. Extensive preoperative diagnostic (in particular in 2 descensus cases) would have been appropriate here. The one iatrogenic injury (ureter ligature, 471/0) in this group has only played a secondary role with the purulent pyelonephritis and hydronephrosis already present.

Other Causes. We content ourselves with listing the 14 'other causes of death' (2.7%): 7 gastrointestinal hemorrhages (6 ulcers, 1 gastric carcinoma), 2 hepatic comas, 2 diabetes mellitus, 1 anemia in retroperitoneal hematoma, 1 gallbladder carcinoma (88/3, 45 days after operation on a descensus). The cause could not be determined with certainty in 1 case.

Evaluation of Individual Causes of Death. Etiologically, the causes of death could be subdivided into four groups: (1) death was caused by the additional disease already known preoperatively; (2) the quantitatively far smaller group of injuries due to the operation; (3) complications which arose postoperatively, and (4) terminal stages of the primary disease operated on. The ways of lowering postoperative mortality are also indicated by this classification.

A significant connection between the age of the patients who died and the individual causes of death could not be demonstrated. Merely the higher mortality rate in cases of bronchopneumonia can be explained by the multimorbidity due to age in the very old patients (8.6% of all deaths and 19.4% of deaths in 80-year-old and older patients operated on).

Table 54 gives information on the postoperative deaths in relation to the time after operation, the average duration of the postoperative phase and their mean values. With a longer postoperative phase, a direct connection between the operation and exitus becomes ever less probable. It is thus not astonishing that the 'immediate mortality' (mostly a consequence of the inadequate treatment of postoperative shock) displaces the shortest postoperative duration. A possible connection with the intervention is to be assumed in the causes of death with low mean values: ileus (6.6 days), peritonitis (7.1 days), bronchopneumonia (8.3 days) and 'cardiovascular failure' (8.8 days). Then follow pulmonary embolism with 10.8 days and 'other causes of death' with 13.0 days.

The median values of 15.5 days in kidney failure and 23.9 days in organic diseases of the cardiovascular system might be evaluated as an indication for the

Table 55. Postoperative mortality in disease groups

Disease group	Total cases	Exitus			autopsy	
		cases	%		cases	%
			in disease group	of those who died		
Genital displacements	1,993	40	2.0	7.8	20	50.0
Malignant tumors	3,111	377	12.1	74.0	206	54.5
Benign tumors	1,141	57	5.0	11.2	37	64.9
Other gynecological diseases	266	17	6.0	3.1	7	43.8
Other surgical diseases	147	20	13.6	3.9	12	60.0
Total	6,658	511	7.7	100.0	282	55.2

multimorbidity which was already present preoperatively in the patients who die postoperatively. By far the longest average duration of treatment (49.1 days with the median value of 44.6 days) are shown by the patients with malignancies who died of 'tumor cachexia'. Nevertheless, 17 women die in the first 14 days after the operation: an ovarian carcinoma was involved 9 times (5 exploratory laparotomies, 3 emergency laparotomies and 1 tumor extirpation), a collum carcinoma was involved 4 times (3 exploratory laparotomies and 1 abdominal hysterectomy), a corpus carcinoma was involved twice (both exploratory laparotomies) and an exploratory laparotomy in a gallbladder carcinoma was involved once. A patient with breast cancer (1121/0) died with the diagnosis of a tumor cachexia on the 12th day after operation. Especially in the patients who died so early, the question arises as to whether the intervention was reasonably indicated. This question cannot be answered retrospectively. The high proportion of exploratory laparotomies is noticeable here.

Kind of Disease and Postoperative Mortality

We recorded the highest postoperative mortality (13.6%) in other surgical diseases. The malignant tumors follow with 12.1%. In the other disease groups, the mortality was very much lower: in other gynecological diseases 6.0%, in benign tumors 5.0% and in genital displacements 2.0% (table 55).

The 377 patients with malignancies who die postoperatively amount to 74.0% of the total postoperative mortality. The 57 women who died with benign genital tumors constitute 11.2% of all deaths and the 40 women who died with

Table 56. Causes of death in disease groups

Disease group	Total	'Immediate mortality'	'Cardiovascular failure'	Organic diseases of cardiovascular system	Pulmonary embolism	Broncho-pneumonia	Kidney failure	Peritonitis	Ileus	Tumor cachexia	Other causes
Genital displacements	40 7.8%	1 2.5% 4.0%	3 7.5% 2.9%	8 20.0% 22.9%	18 45.0% 20.0%	4 10.0% 9.1%	2 5.0% 11.1%	2 5.0% 2.8%	0	0	2 5.0% 14.3%
Malignant tumors	377 73.8%	18 4.8% 72.0%	82 21.8% 79.6%	22 5.8% 62.9%	52 13.8% 57.8%	37 9.8% 84.1%	11 2.9% 61.1%	49 13.0% 68.1%	22 5.8% 62.9%	75 19.9% 100.0%	9 2.4% 64.3%
Benign tumors	57 11.2%	5 8.8% 20.0%	12 21.1% 11.7%	4 7.0% 11.4%	15 26.3% 16.7%	1 1.8% 2.3%	2 3.5% 11.1%	7 12.3% 9.7%	9 15.8% 25.7%	0	2 3.5% 14.3%
Other gynecological diseases	17 3.3%	1 5.9% 4.0%	4 23.5% 3.9%	1 5.9% 2.9%	1 5.9% 1.1%	2 11.8% 4.5%	2 11.8% 11.1%	4 23.5% 5.6%	2 11.8% 5.7%	0	0
Other surgical diseases	20 3.9%	0	2 10.0% 1.9%	0	4 20.0% 4.4%	0	1 5.0% 5.6%	10 50.0% 13.9%	2 10.0% 5.7%	0	1 5.0% 7.1%
Total	511 100.0%	25 4.9%	103 20.2%	35 6.8%	90 17.6%	44 8.6%	18 3.5%	72 14.1%	35 6.8%	75 14.7%	14 2.7%

genital displacements 7.8%. In consequence of the low absolute numbers, the 20 deaths in women with other surgical diseases make up only 3.9% of the total postoperative mortality. 17 patients who died with other gynecological diseases make up 3.1% of the total mortality. In the first 14 days after operation, 317 women died (62.0%). In the genital displacements, there were 19 patients (47.5%), and in the malignancies 226 patients (59.9%). Of 57 deaths in benign tumors, 40 (70.1%) took place in the first 2 weeks after the intervention. We recorded the greatest mortality rate in this period with 88.2% (15 out of 17 fatalities) in other gynecological diseases. The other surgical diseases also display a high postoperative fatality of 85.0% (17 out of 20 deaths). Here the not always adequate preoperative preparation of the patients mostly operated on under assumption of an ovarian tumor has probably played a role.

Table 56 gives a survey of the causes of death in the disease groups. The first row of the percentage figures gives the proportions of all causes of death in the individual disease groups, and the second row gives the proportion of individual causes of death in all disease groups.

Malignant Tumors

The relative frequency of the causes of death in various malignant tumors in the individual age groups (e.g. exitus in collum and ovarian carcinomas are more frequent in the first, and exitus in corpus and mammary carcinoma are more frequent in the last age group) exclusively depends on the absolute number of the specified tumors (table 57). The causes of death specified in the patients who died with malignancies are listed in table 58. However, just like some differences in the average postoperative duration, they are first discussed in the section on individual tumors.

Vulvar and Vaginal Carcinoma. The 87 cases of vulvar carcinomas are in our opinion burdened with a too high postoperative mortality of 6.9%. Of 6 patients who died, only 1 was autopsied. Thus the 4 fatalities in the first 2 postoperative weeks after a vulvectomy could not be explained by a pathological anatomical finding:

Case 967/0: 73-year-old patient, pulseless on the 8th day after operation, cardiac massage, 'cardiovascular failure'.

Case 339/2: 80-year-old patient, operation on the day of admission. Among the symptoms a pulmonary embolism, exitus on the 3rd postoperative day. Autopsy refused.

Case 122/4: 72-year-old patient, operation without previous digitalization, 'acute cardiac arrest'.

Case 134/4: Pulmonary embolism verified by autopsy on the 7th day after operation.

The only case of death after operation on a vaginal carcinoma (104/9) was caused by septicopyemia and peritonitis after abdominal hysterectomy with vaginal cuff.

Table 57. Postoperative mortality in malignant diseases

Localization of malignancy	Total cases	Exitus			autopsy	
		cases	%		cases	%
			in disease group	of those who died		
Vulva	87	6	6.9	1.6	1	16.7
Vagina	15	1	6.7	0.3	1	100.0
Uterine cervix	326	40	12.3	10.6	26	65.0
Corpus uteri	763	72	9.4	19.1	44	61.1
Tube	29	8	27.6	2.1	6	75.0
Ovary	604	150	24.8	39.8	75	50.0
General carcinosis	37	9	24.3	2.4	1	11.1
Extragenital intraperitoneal	106	55	51.9	14.6	30	54.5
Extraperitoneal	19	8	42.1	2.1	8	100.0
Breast	1,125	28	2.5	7.4	14	50.0
Total	3,111	377	12.1	100.0	206	54.5

Collum Carcinoma. In 326 operations on the collum carcinoma, we recorded a postoperative mortality of 12.3% with 40 deaths (table 59). This figure is influenced by 18 deaths (54.5%) in 33 emergency laparotomies. The palliative laparotomies and exploratory laparotomies also burden the postoperative lethality in this malignancy. The low mortality rates after radical vaginal and abdominal operations (2.1 and 8.3%, respectively) are worth mentioning. They prove that age is no contraindication to surgery. Vaginal hysterectomy constitutes an incomplete surgical method in collum carcinoma. Thus 19 of these interventions without subsequent exitus are not relevant.

Corpus Carcinoma. Of 763 patients operated on, 72 (9.4%) died after the intervention. Table 59 shows that 8 palliative laparotomies (27.6%), 15 exploratory laparotomies (50.0%) and 3 emergency laparotomies (42.9%) contribute considerably to the postoperatively lethality. The 36 deaths in 477 abdominal hysterectomies correspond to a postoperative mortality of 7.5%.

Tubal Carcinoma. We have recorded 29 tubal carcinomas which were operated on. The 8 patients who died (27.6%) are an indication of the advanced stage (for details, see p. 99).

Table 58. Causes of death in some malignancies

Localization of malignancy	Total cases	'Immediate mortality'	'Cardiovascular failure'	Organic diseases of cardiovascular system	Pulmonary embolism	Bronchopneumonia	Kidney failure	Peritonitis	Ileus	Tumor cachexia	Other causes
Vulva	6	1	2	–	2	–	–	–	–	1	–
Vagina	1	–	–	–	–	–	–	1	–	–	–
Uterine cervix	40	2	2	1	5	3	4	9	1	12	1
Corpus uteri	72	5	11	8	17	7	2	6	5	6	5
Tube	8	–	1	–	3	2	–	1	–	1	–
Ovary	150	6	41	6	15	18	4	15	11	33	1
General carcinosis	9	1	4	–	1	–	–	–	1	2	–
Extragenital intraperitoneal malignancies	55	1	15	1	6	5	1	14	4	7	1
Extraperitoneal malignancies	8	1	1	1	–	1	–	2	–	2	–
Breast	28	1	5	5	3	1	–	1	–	11	1
Total malignancies	377	18	82	22	52	37	11	49	22	75	9
Total fatalities	511	25	103	35	90	44	18	72	35	75	14

Table 59. Postoperative mortality after operations on some malignancies

Operation	Uterine cervix			Corpus uteri			Ovary		
	cases	exitus		cases	exitus		cases	exitus	
		n	%		n	%		n	%
Schauta's operation	97	2	2.1	6	0	0.0	–	–	–
Vaginal hysterectomy	19	0	0.0	208	9	4.3	–	–	–
Wertheim's operation or evisceration	108	9	8.3	6	1	16.7	2	1	50.0
Abdominal hysterectomy	38	5	13.2	477	36	7.5	191	24	12.4
Palliative laparotomy	21	4	19.0	29	8	27.6	236	50	21.2
Exploratory laparotomy	10	2	20.0	30	15	50.0	156	61	39.1
Emergency laparotomy	33	18	54.5	7	3	42.9	19	14	73.7
Total	326	40	12.3	763	72	9.4	604	150	24.8

Ovarian Carcinoma. Of 604 patients with a malignant ovarian tumor, 150 died after the operation (24.8%). The mortality in individual interventions greatly depends on the extent of ovarian cancer (table 59). We cannot be satisfied that 1 woman in 4 died after the operation. We have pointed out some possibilities of improving this unsatisfactory situation on page 104.

General Carcinosis. In 37 cases of general carcinosis, 9 deaths are recorded, corresponding to a postoperative mortality of 24.3%. 8 patients who died were not autopsied. That there was no autopsy to clarify the primary localization of the malignancy is especially regrettable here. We recorded a further 25 cases in which the surgical intervention was terminated with a diagnosis of a 'general carcinosis'; in these cases, the primary localization of the underlying disease could be found at autopsy.

Extragenital Intraperitoneal Malignancies. The 106 extragenital intraperitoneal malignancy operations are burdened with 55 deaths. These largely concern patients with tumors of the gastrointestinal tract. The mortality was 41% after operations on rectal-sigmoid carcinomas (68 cases), 75% in the colon malignancies, and even 100% in 7 gallbladder carcinomas. This figure shows that the great extent of the process has primarily contributed to exitus and less the kind and extent of the intervention (exploratory laparotomy 4 times, salpingo-oophorectomy twice and abdominal hysterectomy with adnexae once). The postoperative mortality is high (51.9%), and only the small number of cases keeps the negative influence on the total postoperative lethality within limits. The necessity of complete preoperative diagnostics before laparotomy is thereby proved once more.

Retroperitoneal Malignancies. In this group, we have registered 8 deaths out of a total of 19 operations (42.1%). They are to be assessed like the extragenital, intraperitoneal malignancies.

Breast Cancer. In our breast cancer patients there were 28 deaths (2.5%), representing the lowest postoperative mortality of all malignancies. The hypothesis can be postulated that the premature exitus might have been avoided by a primary irradiation, especially in elderly patients. Only a detailed analysis of the postoperative mortality can decide whether surgical treatment of breast cancer is justified in elderly women. The breast cancer patients died at a significantly greater time interval from the intervention compared to other cancer patients. We registered 15 deaths (53.5%) after the 29th postoperative day.

In 28 deaths, autopsy was not performed 14 times (50%). In 7 out of 11 cases with tumor cachexia, in all 5 cases of 'cardiovascular failure', in 1 death (554/3), the clinically diagnosed bronchopneumonia could not be verified because of the refusal of autopsy, and finally autopsy was refrained from in 1 patient (143/8) with recurrent apoplexy. We were unable to detect a direct connection between the fatal pulmonary embolism and the operation on mammary carcinoma in the 3 women who died. 2 women died on the 31st and 51st postoperative day, and in the third patient (146/12), an occlusion of the left 'lower leg vessels' was already diagnosed and treated before her death on the 37th day after operation. 1 patient (127/14) died on the 14th day from a E. coli-pyoceanus sepsis emanating from the surgical wound. A further (233/0) patient died of a bleeding duodenal ulcer on the 9th day after the operation.

In the 28 patients who died, 10 radical mastectomies and 18 ablations were performed. A link between the extent of the intervention and the occurrence of death could not be detected. A correlation is more likely to have existed between the stage of the malignancy and some causes of death.

The question must remain unanswered as to whether the surgical procedure was indicated in 5 breast cancer patients with an organic cardiovascular condition (573/0: Adams-Stokes attacks; 24/12: decompensated hypertension; 22/14: coronary sclerosis in arterial hypertension; 143/8: recurrent apoplexy; 150/12: chronic cardiac insufficiency, pulmonary emphysema and now hemiplegia), and to what extent the operation as such has critically worsened the cardiovascular disease situation.

In the 11 cases of tumor cachexia, the question had to be posed as to whether the extent of the underlying disease was correctly assessed preoperatively in all women who died up to the 94th postoperative day. The same also applies to the 5 cases of cardiovascular failure which were not autopsied: for example, in case 37/15, a pleural effusion was known, the patient died 8 days after an ablatio mammae. Despite some cases with perhaps avoidable lethal outcome, surgical treatment of mammary carcinoma remains the method of choice, even in elderly women.

The mortality rate does not differ between the individual gynecology departments. A slight exception is the gynecology department 15: among 86 interventions, an operation on a malignancy was involved 46 times. Out of 20 breast cancer patients, 4 (20%) died of cardiovascular failure which were not verified by autopsy.

Benign Tumors

There is a different situation in the analysis of postoperative mortality after operations on benign tumors. Postoperative histological investigation is also indispensable in these tumors for clarification of the cancer risk.

In 57 deaths, patients with a benign ovarian tumor were involved 46 times (80.7%). Table 51 shows the postoperative mortality after individual operations. The low lethality after abdominal hysterectomies with adnexae shows that this operation does not constitute an exceptional strain for the patients when carried out consistently. In 193 operations on a uterus myomatosus, we have registered 8 postoperative deaths (the women died in 4.1% of all uterus myomatosus operations and 14.0% died after operation on a benign tumor). There were 5 deaths after 135 hysterectomies (3.7%) and 3 deaths after 41 supravaginal uterine amputations (7.3%). The small absolute values do not admit any statistically significant statement. They can be interpreted as in the ovarian tumors. There remain 3 deaths to analyze which only partially belong here.

Case 223/9: A 67-year-old patient was laparotomized under the assumption of an ovarian tumor. It was in fact a hemorrhagic splenic tumor in existing leukemia. The patient died of peritonitis after splenectomy.

Case 121/1: There was ureter cyst. The patient died of a sepsis.

Case 485/1: The suspected ovarian tumor proved to be a hydronephrosis. The patient did not survive a postoperative shock.

Other Gynecological Diseases

In 17 other gynecological diseases with fatal course, 4 deaths in cases of inflammatory genital processes are described.

Case 336/5: Suspicion of an ovarian tumor was not confirmed at laparotomy. Adhesiolysis in a conglomerate tumor. Cause of death: 'cardiovascular failure' (fecal fistula of the small intestine at autopsy).

Case 212/8: Adnexal conglomerate tumor, salpingo-oophorectomy with adhesiolysis. Cause of death: sigmoid fistula, fecal peritonitis.

Case 22/6: Pyosalpinx. Salpingo-oophorectomy in existing anuria. Cause of death: kidney failure.

Table 60. Causes of death in operations on genital displacements

Kind of operation	Total cases	Fatalities			'immediate mortality'	'cardiovascular failure'	organic disease of cardiovascular system	pulmonary embolism	broncho-pneumonia	kidney failure	perito-nitis	other causes
		cases	% in kind of operation	% of all fatalities								
Vaginal hysterectomy	419	3	0.7	7.5	1	–	1	1	–	–	–	–
Portio amputation	205	3	1.5	7.5	–	–	–	3	–	–	–	–
Anterior and posterior colporrhaphies	495	13	2.6	32.5	–	1	3	7	1	1	–	–
Posterior colporrhaphy	137	1	0.7	2.5	–	–	–	–	1	–	–	–
Semicolpocleisis (Labhardt's operation)	243	9	3.7	22.5	–	1	2	2	1	1	–	2
Colpoepisiocleisis (Conill's operation)	28	2	7.1	5.0	–	–	1	1	–	–	–	–
Semicolpocleisis (Neugebauer-LeFort's operation)	215	7	3.3	17.5	–	1	1	3	1	–	1	–
Abdominal stump extirpation	2	1	50.0	2.5	–	–	–	–	–	–	1	–
Uterus fixation (Doléris' operation)	22	1	4.5	2.5	–	–	–	1	–	–	–	–
Other operations	227	–	–	–	–	–	–	–	–	–	–	–
Total	1,993	40	2.0	100.0	1	3	8	18	4	2	2	2
%					2.5	7.5	20.0	45.0	10	5	5	5

Case 7/9: Pyometra. Abdominal hysterectomy with adnexae. Cause of death: 'cardiovascular failure'.

Of 15 women operated on for a uterine perforation, 3 died.

Case 375/2: Condition after perforation and abdominal hysterectomy at another hospital. Admission with sepsis. Only intestinal fistulation possible as therapy. Cause of death: 'cardiovascular failure'.
Case 399/4: Uterine perforation external, merely Douglas drainage. Cause of death: peritonitis.
Case 332/9: The uterine perforation was treated properly by abdominal hysterectomy. The patient died of the consequences of a visceral eventration.

In 3 urogenital fistulae, the terminal stage of a malignancy was involved twice (249/1, 326/1) and a condition after Wertheim operation once (261/2). The patient died on the 8th postoperative day after a Boari operation. Cause of death: suture insufficiency, phlegmon in the retroperitoneal space.

In the other patients who died, we found the following indications for surgery: recurrent metrorrhagia (591/2), carcinoma in situ (448/3), suspect portio (141/4), 'suspicion of corpus carcinoma' (101/107), abdominal wall operation because of a pendulous abdomen (55/3). The putative diagnosis 'ovarian tumor' could not be confirmed at laparotomy in 2 cases (235/0, 285/5).

Other Surgical Conditions

Of 20 deaths, 15 women with a sigmoid diverticulitis are to be mentioned. We have already discussed the problems in differential diagnosis of this disease. 3 out of 4 women who died from an appendicitis or from a perityphlitic abscess were operated on under the assumption of an ovarian tumor. A 65-year-old patient (466/0) died of peritonitis after correction of a scar hernia.

Genital Displacements

The 40 postoperative deaths constitute only 2.0% of all descensus and prolapse operations and 7.8% of all deaths. However, they are far more serious than in all other disease groups. We must always bear in mind here that the patients who die might perhaps have lived for several years more without the operation. In a mortality which is too high, the justification of the extended gynecological indication for surgery at an advanced age must indeed be placed in doubt. A careful assessment of the indications taking into account the possible postoperative complications is indispensable in precisely these patients.

In table 60 is found the evaluation of the kind of operation and the causes of death. The individual interventions are burdened with different mortality rates. These depend on other factors than the kind of operation. Nevertheless, we should like to mention the 3 postoperative deaths after 419 vaginal hysterectomies with colporrhaphies. They correspond to a mortality of 0.7%, which must be regarded as positive. It justifies recommendation of vaginal hysterectomy with colporrhaphies as the surgical method of choice for treatment of descensus and prolapse, even in old women.

Analysis of individual causes of death has crucial importance. Another distribution is seen here than in all deaths together: on the one hand, there is no tumor cachexia or ileus, and on the other hand there is a more frequent relative and absolute occurrence of pulmonary embolism (45%) and organic cardiovascular diseases (20%).

Of 18 cases of pulmonary embolism, 13 were verified by autopsy. The clinical symptoms were sufficient for this diagnosis 5 times. The women died under the picture of cerebral apoplexy in 5 cases (429/1, 8/2, 155/5, 87/8); the cerebral bleeding was verified by autopsy only once (163/9). A 70-year-old patient (68/4) died after a semicolpocleisis on the 33rd day after operation. The autopsy revealed a ventricular insufficiency with final dilatation. The diagnosis of 2 myocardial infarctions (236/8, 128/11) was based on the clinical symptoms or ECG and laboratory findings. Autopsies were not ordered.

This also applies to all 4 cases of bronchopneumonia. A connection with the intervention is to be assumed in 2 cases, since the patients (55/7, 54/15) died on the 6th and 7th postoperative day. This connection appears doubtful in a patient (44/10) who died 36 days after the intervention. The bronchopneumonia with fatal outcome in the 4th case (485/5) is not causally related to the semicolpocleisis performed; exitus occurred 104 days after the operation. The 3 cases of 'cardiovascular failure' (616/0, 685/1, 35/5) make up only 7.5% of all deaths. This diagnosis is evidently often avoided in benign conditions.

Infection in the abdomen was stated as the cause of death in 2 cases.

Case 266/2: Condition after supravaginal uterine amputation with portio fixation, recurrence of descensus. Now abdominal stump extirpation with colporrhaphies. On the 17th day after operation, exitus 2 h after surgical attention to the visceral eventration.

Case 63/8: Descensus, vaginal hysterectomy with colporrhaphies. Exitus on the 8th day after operation. At autopsy a peritonitis in consequence of severe purulent cholecystitis was found.

Case 301/7: A 61-year-old obese diabetic with posterior vaginal hernia and rectocele died on the 26th day after a Labhardt semicolpocleisis. Cause of death: urosepsis.

Case 530/0: Vaginal descensus in a 64-year-old patient with hernia known for 20 years. Colporrhaphies and herniotomy. 12 days after the operation hematuria (therefore cystoscopy, no note on its being performed before the operation): blood and pus comes from the right ureter. Exitus on the 23rd day after operation. Autopsy: severe destructive pyelonephritis.

We are able to assign one exitus to the group of 'immediate mortality': a 62-year-old diabetic (95/2) with descensus died on the day of operation after a vaginal hysterectomy with adnexae and colporrhaphies. Autopsy: 'central respiratory arrest'. Finally, 2 case records belong to the 'other causes of death'.

Case 425/5: A 67-year-old patient died 12 days after a semicolpocleisis with hematemesis which could not be stopped. Although a uremic coma was also stated, there was no autopsy.

Case 88/3: A 61-year-old patient died 54 days after a Labhardt semicolpocleisis. A gallbladder carcinoma was found as the cause of death at autopsy.

Retrospectively, some deaths appear to have been avoidable. With more extensive preoperative diagnostics, one could probably have dispensed with surgical corrections of the genital displacements. The high proportion of pulmonary embolism likewise shows possibilities for reducing the postoperative mortality after descensus and prolapse operations. According to this analysis, we believe we can assert that in spite of the regrettable deaths the positive attitude to surgical treatment of genital displacements remains justified.

Kind of Operation and Postoperative Mortality

Table 61 gives us an overview of the postoperative mortality in the individual kinds of operation. The very great differences are only interpreted later on page 141. At this point, only very much higher postoperative mortality after

Table 61. Postoperative mortality in individual kinds of operation

Kind of operation	Total cases	Exitus			autopsy	
		cases	%			
			in operation group	of those who died	cases	%
Vulva operations	121	6	5.0	1.2	1	16.7
Vaginal operations on the descensus	1,174	24	2.0	4.7	13	54.2
Vaginal operations on uterine prolapse	695	14	2.0	2.7	6	42.9
Abdominovaginal descensus/prolapse operations	124	1	1.6	0.4	1	50.0
Vaginal operations	468	13	2.7	2.5	9	69.2
'Total' gynecological laparotomies	2,042	146	7.1	28.6	87	59.6
Gynecological palliative, exploratory, emergency laparotomies	621	192	30.9	37.6	98	51.0
'Total' surgical laparotomies	171	34	19.8	6.7	23	67.6
Surgical palliative, exploratory, and emergency laparotomies	117	52	44.4	10.1	30	57.7
Breast operations	1,125	28	2.5	5.5	14	50.0
Total	6,658	511	7.7	100.0	282	55.2

Table 62. Postoperative mortality in laparotomies

Kind of laparotomy	Total cases	Exitus				autopsy	
		cases	%				
			in kind of laparotomy	of those who died		cases	%
'Complete' gynecological laparotomies	2,042	146	7.1	34.4		87	59.6
Gynecological palliative laparotomies	297	64	21.5	15.1		29	45.3
Gynecological exploratory laparotomies	249	90	36.1	21.2		45	50.0
Gynecological emergency laparotomies	75	38	51.4	9.1		24	63.2
'Complete' surgical laparotomies	171	34	19.8	68.0		23	67.6
Surgical palliative laparotomies	12	4	33.3	0.9		3	75.0
Surgical exploratory laparotomies	88	40	45.5	9.4		24	60.0
Surgical emergency laparotomies	17	8	47.1	1.9		3	37.5
Total laparotomies	2,955	424	14,3	100,0		238	56,1
Total interventions	6,658	511	7,7			282	55,2

the laparotomies will be analyzed. The data in table 62 serve for this purpose. The highest mortality is found in gynecological emergency laparotomies (51.4%) and in surgical emergency laparotomies (47.1%). Of 249 gynecological exploratory laparotomies, 90 (36.1%) ended lethally and of 88 surgical exploratory laparotomies 40 (45.5%) ended lethally. The kind of operation which is gentlest in terms of extent and duration is burdened with a very much larger postoperative mortality in our material than is complete laparotomy (7.3 or 19.9%). Just as serious is the observation that the 130 deaths in exploratory laparotomies amount to 25.4% of all deaths and 30.6% of the deaths in laparotomies. This justifies a search for the causes of such a high mortality and for possibilities of reducing it.

120 women who died after an exploratory laparotomy (92.3%) suffered from a malignancy which was no longer operable. The predominance of the ovarian carcinoma is pointed out once more in this context. In the 10 inflammatory processes (3 of gynecological and 7 of surgical origin), almost always fateful attempts at adhesiolysis are made. We have already pointed out how dangerous they are, especially in inflammatory intestinal conditions (198).

We see three possibilities of reducing the numbers of exploratory laparotomies:

(1) General intensification of preventive examinations in elderly women. These investigations do not only consist in preparing a smear according to

Table 63. Causes of death in individual kind of operation

Kind of operation	Total cases	'Immediate mortality'	'Cardiovascular failure'	Organic diseases of cardiovascular system	Pulmonary embolism	Broncho-pneumonia	Kidney failure	Peritonitis	Ileus	Tumor cachexia	Other causes
Vulva operations	6	1	2	–	2	–	–	–	–	1	–
Vaginal operations on descensus	24	1	2	3	11	3	2	–	–	–	2
Vaginal operations on uterine prolapse	14	–	1	5	6	1	–	1	–	–	–
Abdominovaginal descensus/prolapse operations	2	–	–	–	1	–	–	1	–	–	1
Vaginal operations	13	1	–	1	5	2	–	3	–	–	1
'Complete' gynecological laparotomies	146	10	26	15	28	14	7	17	17	6	6
Gynecological palliative, exploratory, and emergency laparotomies	192	8	49	4	24	17	7	21	12	48	2
'Complete' surgical laparotomies	34	2	4	–	4	3	–	14	3	3	1
Surgical palliative, exploratory, and emergency laparotomies	52	1	14	2	6	3	2	14	3	6	1
Breast operations	28	1	5	5	3	1	–	1	–	11	–
Total	511	25	103	35	90	44	18	72	35	75	14

Table 64. Causes of death in individual laparotomies

Kind of laparotomy	Total cases	'Immediate mortality'	'Cardiovascular failure'	Organic diseases of cardiovascular system	Pulmonary embolism	Bronchopneumonia	Kidney failure	Peritonitis	Ileus	Tumor cachexia	Other causes
'Complete' gynecological laparotomies	146	10	26	15	28	14	7	17	17	6	6
Gynecological palliative laparotomies	64	6	23	1	6	7	1	11	3	6	–
Gynecological exploratory laparotomies	90	2	23	1	18	8	2	5	7	22	2
Gynecological emergency laparotomies	38	–	3	2	–	2	4	5	2	20	–
'Complete' surgical laparotomies	34	2	4	–	4	3	–	14	3	3	1
Surgical palliative laparotomies	4	1	–	1	–	–	–	1	–	1	–
Surgical exploratory laparotomies	40	–	11	1	6	2	2	10	3	4	1
Surgical emergency laparotomies	8	–	3	–	–	1	–	3	–	1	–
Total laparotomies	424	21	93	21	62	37	16	66	35	63	10
Total interventions	511	25	103	35	90	44	18	72	35	75	14

Papanicolaou, but also in careful palpation. Gynecological cancer prevention should therefore be exclusively reserved to the specialist doctors. It is primarily a matter of detecting the incipient (still operable) malignant processes. Large ovarian tumors are often not noticed by the patients themselves.

(2) Complete preoperative diagnostics. Comprehensive preoperative diagnostics (including the performance of a colon contrast enema) may indicate sigmoid diverticulitis. Outpatient diagnostics with subsequent fractionated abrasion or conization would very probably give an indication for the presence of a collum carcinoma in appropriate cases.

(3) Application of laparoscopy (see p. 142).

There is no connection between the kind of operation and the age of patients who died. A correlation also cannot be found between the time of death and the method of operation. The clustering of the deaths after a vulvectomy in the first postoperative weeks is coincidental. The displacement of the deaths in time after prolapse and breast operations is to be explained by the underlying disease and the causes of death.

Table 63 (intentionally without percentages) gives us an overview of the causes of death in the individual kinds of operation. The vaginal operations are hardly burdened by particular causes of death, e.g. ileus or peritonitis. The causes of death in laparotomies are listed in table 64. 'Tumor cachexia' is found especially in exploratory and emergency gynecological laparotomies.

Evaluation of the Postoperative Mortality

Although we have refrained from any statistical rectification, the postoperative mortality (7.7%) still suggests some alternatives for lowering it: (1) various possibilities in individual cases (only a few examples are named), and (2) improvement of postoperative attention and treatment.

(1a) Avoidance of non-specific and inadequate exploratory excisions:

Case 363/0: In 1961 condyloma acumina, January 1964 papilloma vulvae, April 1964 carcinoma vulvae.
Case 253/3: Exploratory excision from an urethral ectropion in colporrhaphies: benign; 1 year later fresh exploratory excision: urethral carcinoma.
Case 86/9: On August 7, 1962, stomach operation with benign histological finding. On November 14, 1962, abdominal hysterectomy with adnexae and omental resection because of a multolocular pseudomucinous ovarian tumor. Exitus 3 days later. Autopsy: gastric carcinoma with bleeding.
Case 109/5: General carcinomatosis, exploratory laparotomy, exploratory excision: merely adipose and connective tissue. No autopsy after exitus.

All cases of exploratory laparotomies without biopsies are to be evaluated similarly (e.g. 259/5, 285/5).

(1b) Timely termination of the objective palpatory finding:

Case 191/8: On July 3, 1967, benign histological finding of an abradate with normal palpatory finding. On August 16, 1967, bilateral ovariectomy with an ovarian carcinoma filling the entire pelvis. Exitus on August 31, 1967.

Case 246/6: An external abrasion 4 weeks ago because of metrorrhagias; now an extensive ovarian carcinoma necessitates application of an anus praeter.

Case 82/15: In February and April, two descensus operations, in September, exitus from metastatic ovarian carcinoma.

(1c) Adequate preoperative preparation:

Case 339/2: Hemivulvectomy on the day of admission in an 80-year-old patient. Exitus on the 3rd postoperative day in consequence of arrhythmias.

(1d) Complete preoperative diagnostics:

Case 471/0: 'The parts of the uterus affected by the sarcoma can be removed without preparing out the ureter.' Exitus on the 16th day after operation. Autopsy: kidney failure, purulent pyelonephritis on both sides, bilateral hydronephrosis, ureterolith occlusion on the right, ligature of the left ureter.

(1e) Optimal indication for intervention:

Case 64/9: Collum carcinoma, Volhard test, but no intravenous pyelogram. RR 210/130 mm Hg. The surgical intervention was kept as small as possible: supravaginal uterine amputation with adnexae. Exitus shortly afterwards. Autopsy: bilateral hydronephrosis and hydroureter.

(1f) In indicated cases, laparoscopy is to be aimed for instead of a primary laparotomy where the patient is prepared to undergo laparotomy.

(2) The 317 deaths within the first 14 postoperative days constitute 62.0% of the total postoperative mortality. This clearly points to the central concern of our efforts to lower the postoperative mortality, namely the necessity of complex prevention and intensive treatment of postoperative complications.

In contrast to the period of the report, anesthesia is carried out as a rule by anesthesists. These mostly have several techniques available and are able to recognize and treat intraoperative cardiac, circulatory and pulmonary complications better. Suitable anesthetic techniques enable side effects on damaged patients to be avoided (e.g. no uncontrolled anesthesia such as PDA or barbiturate monoanesthesia in shock patients). The demand for intensive postoperative care has been taken into account in the meantime with the establishment of special wards for patients recovering from anesthesia and intensive wards. The co-operation of the gynecologist with the anesthesists is thus not limited to the short time of the operation, but extends to the immediate postoperative phase, and if necessary also beyond this. Through the recognition of dangerous postoperative complications (hemorrhage, shock, respiratory insufficiency, kidney failure) and its immediate intensive treatment, the postoperative mortality can be lowered. The question remains open as to whether the mortality is only shifted from the early into the late phase (more dependent on nursing measures and the general condition of the patients), or whether the total mortality in fact falls.

The 90 cases of pulmonary embolism show that their prophylaxis before and after the intervention has not lost any topicality, and that pulmonary embolism in geriatric gynecological operation cases has remained as therapeutic problem of first priority. The 44 bronchopneumonias show the importance of intensive postoperative physiotherapy, especially after geriatric operations. The organic cardiovascular diseases leading to death show the importance of the presence of multimorbidity. In principle, this should not constitute a contraindication to intervention, e.g. in justified suspicion of a gynecological malignancy. The postoperative cerebral thromboembolic complication underscore the demands already made in pulmonary embolism. In 72 peritonitis cases and 35 cases of ileus, we got the impression that the treatment of these serious postoperative complications has not always been prosecuted with due intensity. We mean in particular the small number of relaparotomies.

Individual Clinical Problems

Route of Surgery in Individual Diseases

Muth (241) and *Terzi et al.* (300) compared the postoperative mortality after vaginal and abdominal procedure and recommend that more attention be given to the vaginal approach. According to *Stožický and Vácha* (291), vaginal interventions should be given preference in cases with raised risk of surgery. We should like to examine the practical applicability of these views by analyzing our own material.

Out of 1,993 cases of genital displacements, 1,869 (93.8%) were operated on vaginally. In the 124 'abdominal-vaginal' or 'abdominal' operations, we must (as already mentioned) criticize only 22 cases of Doléris' antefixation of the uterus or Kocher's exohysteropexy. In 3,111 malignant tumors, only one 'route of operation' was possible from the beginning in 2,022 cases (65.1%): 87 vulva carcinomas, 15 vaginal carcinomas, 29 tubal carcinomas, 604 ovarian carcinomas, 37 general carcinoses, 106 extragenital intraperitoneal malignancies, 19 extraperitoneal malignances and 1,125 mammary carcinomas.

With appropriate indication, both the vaginal and the abdominal route are reserved only for collum and corpus carcinomas. The 108 Wertheim operations in collum carcinoma and the 477 abdominal hysterectomies in corpus carcinoma constitute merely 18.8% of all malignancy operations. It must be taken into account here that the conditions for the vaginal procedure were not always favorable (e.g., the patients had not had a pregnancy, uterus myomatosus, additional adnexal finding).

We should like to limit the statement of *Randow and Riess* (263) on vaginal hysterectomy in corpus carcinomas in one point: the adnexae must be removed along with the uterus in every corpus carcinoma even with a vaginal procedure because of the known metastasis (in our patients, this took place in only 156 out of 216 cases); if technical difficulties in surgery are expected, abdominal hysterectomy with bilateral salpingo-oophorectomy must be chosen. In 1,141 benign genital tumors, the respective localization decided the kind of operation. The 11 vaginal hysterectomies in uterus myomatosus and in particular the 10 vaginal extirpations of an ovarian tumor must be regarded as an exception. In the 266 other gynecological diseases, the surgical procedure was clear. The 65 cases of a carcinoma in situ were operated on 31 times abdominally and 34 times vaginally. In 44 cases a recurrent bleeding without other pathological gynecological findings, the uterus was removed abdominally 20 times and vaginally 24 times.

The advantages of the vaginal procedure compared to laparotomy are sufficiently known and also fully taken into account in the treatment of patients in West Berlin gynecology departments. The cases with fatal outcome after laparotomy could not have been operated on vaginally. Thus, no recommendation in favor of the one or the other procedure can be derived from the dissimilar postoperative mortality in vaginal and abdominal operations.

Ultrasound, Computer Tomography and Laparoscopy in Geriatric Gynecology

Despite the increase of gynecological operations at an advanced age, our most important concern will not be to increase the frequency of operation. The diagnostic use of ultrasound, computer tomography and laparoscopy enable geriatric gynecological laparotomies to be avoided in many cases. In the period which we investigated (1960–1969) these methods were not yet in use. The material in table 65 gives an opportunity to reflect on the avoidability of laparotomies.

Ultrasound investigation is an accessory method for differential diagnosis. It enables an uterus myomatosus to be distinguished from an ovarian tumor (here with great certainty) as well as enabling a tumorous gynecological process to be eliminated indirectly by a negative ultrasound finding.

Access to the diagnostic method of computer tomography will remain difficult for all hospitals, even in the future. Our experience with it is promising, but is not yet sufficient for a publication.

We do not wish to question the principle that every palpable tumor in the true pelvis should be dealt with surgically. The clinical symptoms, e.g. decrease in weight, increase in circumference of the abdomen, ascites (possibly with

Table 65. Possibilities of dispensing with gynecological laparotomy in geriatric operation material

Kind of disease	Total cases	Possible obviation of gynecological laparotomy by laparoscopy		
		cases	no laparotomy	surgical laparotomy
Genital displacements	1,993	–	–	–
Malignant tumors	3,111	356	231	125
Uterine cervix	326	10	10	–
Corpus uteri	763	30	30	–
Tube	29	7	7	–
Ovary	604	156	156	–
General carcinosis	37	28	28	–
Malignant extragenital intraperitoneal tumors	106	106	–	106
Malignant extraperitonal tumors	19	19	–	19
Benign tumors	1,141	16	?	16
Uterine myoma	193	?	?	–
Benign extragenital intraperitoneal tumors	7	7	–	7
Benign extraperitoneal tumors	9	9	–	9
Other gynecological diseases	266	65	65	–
Inflammatory adnexal processes	40	40	40	–
Other gynecological diseases (usually normal genitals)	25	25	25	–
Other surgical diseases	147	113	–	113
Appendicitis	48	48	–	48
Sigmoid diverticulosis, diverticulitis	49	49	–	49
Other surgical diseases	16	16	–	16
Total	6,658	550	296	254

already demonstrated tumor cells) indicates that the operability is restricted in many cases. In our view, a laparoscopy should be considered in all such cases and should be carried out if there is no contraindication and the patient is in agreement. Here we are not only thinking of the lowering of postoperative mortality; rather one can spare many patients the burdensome postoperative phase. Every gynecologist knows cases in which there was no or only a transient improvement of the clinical condition after an exploratory laparotomy and where the intervention only accelerated the lethal outcome.

We have noted three communications on the diagnostic advantages of laparoscopy (196, 200, 322).

Laparoscopy is of importance for surgical geriatric gynecology for two reasons: (1) it enables a good differential diagnosis both between different gynecological diseases and between gynecological and surgical findings, (2) it enables a hitherto indicated laparotomy to be dispensed with. The latter is either not necessary or no longer meaningful. In indicated cases, the surgeon who is already consulted previously can carry out the laparotomy himself.

Portio Stump in Geriatric Surgical Patients

It is of clinical value to determine how high the proportion of women with a portio stump is in our patients. We review on the basis of the diagnoses only 39 cases of a portio stump descensus and 30 cases of a portio stump prolapse. The indication for previous supravaginal uterine amputation was mostly a uterus myomatosus. The cervical stump was removed at the same time in both genital displacements 32 times (46.4%). The surgeons contented themselves 37 times with methods which we believe to be inadequate.

We have registered 74 stump extirpations (56 vaginal, 18 abdominal). The indications for the vaginal interventions were 20 descensus cases, 12 prolapse cases, 9 cervical carcinomas, 2 recurrences of a corpus carinoma and 13 other diseases. The laparotomies involved 2 descensus cases, 8 ovarian tumors, 1 uterine myoma, 2 suspect portios, 1 inflammatory genital condition, 1 recurrent bleeding and 3 collum carcinomas.

We registered 173 supravaginal uterine amputations in our material in 41 cases of uterus myomatosus, 54 benign ovarian tumors, 17 corpus carcinomas, 6 collum carcinomas, 2 tubal carcinomas, 47 ovarian carcinomas, 5 different gynecological diseases and in 1 general carcinosis. We have already described our attitude to this surgical intervention.

Although the number of women with a portio stump after a supravaginal uterine amputation is not large among our patients, we must be concerned to lower the figures still further. This means consistent aiming for complete operation, i.e. hysterectomy (corresponding to the age of the patient with or without adnexae).

Hysterectomy with Both Adnexae as a Standard Geriatric Operation

We have already pointed out the importance of hysterectomy with both adnexae for surgical geriatric gynecology. It appears worthwhile to describe once

Table 66. Proportion of hysterectomies in various gynecological findings

Kind of disease	Total cases	Hysterectomy			
		cases		vaginal	abdominal
		n	%		
Uterine descensus	1,203	204	17.0	198	6
Uterine prolapse	665	226	34.0	221	5
Malignant tumors of vagina	15	3	20.0	2[1]	1
Malignant tumors of uterine cervix	326	205	62.9	97[2]	108[3]
Malignant tumors of corpus uteri	763	697	91.3	214[4]	483[5]
Malignant tumors of tube	29	14	48.3	1	13[6]
Malignant tumors of ovary	604	193	32.0	–	193
General carcinosis	37	4	10.8	–	4
Uterine myoma	193	135	69.9	11	124
Benign ovarian tumors	911	329	36.1	1	328
Pelvic infections	40	17	42.5	1	16
Carcinoma in situ	65	56	86.2	29	27
Uterine bleeding	44	39	88.6	23	16
Perforation of uterus	15	12	80.0	5	7
Suspected portio	12	10	83.3	6	4
Other gynecological diseases	33	7	21.2	3	4

[1] Of these 1 Schauta's operation.
[2] Schauta's operation.
[3] Wertheim's operation.
[4] Of these 6 Schauta's operations.
[5] Of these 6 Wertheim's operations.
[6] Of these 1 Wertheim's operation.

more briefly in table 66 its frequency (in collum carcinoma, the Schauta and Wertheim operations are taken into account).

Many surgical records reveal a certain caution on the part of the surgeons with regard to rather difficult hysterectomies. We regard such reservations as justified only in exceptionally local conditions. For the experienced surgeon, a hysterectomy does not constitute a greater technical problem than supravaginal uterine amputation. In earlier examples of postoperative mortality, an unequivocal extra burden occasioned by abdominal hysterectomy could not be observed. The higher mortality in less invasive operations points rather to the importance of other factors.

According to *Hörmann* (183) the risk of all gynecological operations directly depends on expert assessment of indication and choice of technique, from

intensive individual preparation for operation and from the postoperative follow-up treatment. This principle is absolutely valid for operations in geriatric
gynecology.

Eviscerations in Geriatric Patients

Eviscerations in advanced malignancies in the true pelvis have also been
described in papers on surgical geriatric gynecology (150, 167, 245, 247, 280,
287). *O'Leary and Symmonds* (250) carried out 20 eviscerations in women who
were at least 65 years old. A total eventration was involved 4 times, an anterior
eventration 14 times and a posterior eventration twice. 16 women were 65–69
years old, 3 were 70–74 years old and 1 was more than 75 years old. The
authors have registered 3 deaths after anterior eventration (on the 28th day:
Candida albicans sepsis; on the 13th day: enterocolitis, and on the 41st day
sepsis and insufficient ureterosigmoid anastomosis). Postoperative complications: two ureteroperineal fistulae, a sigmoidovaginal fistula, an enteroperineal
fistula, a rectovaginal fistula, a Douglas abscess and a hematoma in the true
pelvis.

A communication on eviscerations in women of 'geriatric age' was published
by *Noci et al.* (247). 26 collum carcinomas, 3 carcinomas of the body of the
uterus, 1 vaginal carcinoma, 3 sigmoid carcinomas and 1 bladder carcinoma were
involved. These 34 operations constitute 14.1% of all eviscerations carried out in
the gynecology department of the authors. 18 total, 11 anterior and 5 posterior
eviscerations were carried out in 20 60- to 64-year-old, 9 in 65- to 69-year-old
and 5 in 70- to 79-year-old women. The estimation of the risk of surgery is
noteworthy: no raised risk 15 times, moderate risk 17 times, relatively large risk
twice. In no case was there an extreme risk.

In the overall material, the authors registered a postoperative mortality of
37.0%, in geriatric patients the mortality was 32.3%. In 11 patients who died
postoperatively, a collum carcinoma IV was involved 7 times (exitus on the 1st,
3rd, 6th, 8th, 11th, 12th, 16th postoperative day), a collum carcinoma III 3
times (exitus on the 1st, 7th, 8th postoperative day). A patient with sigmoid
carcinoma died on the 5th postoperative day. The causes of death specified
were: 3 cardiovascular decompensations, 3 pulmonary embolisms, 2 peritonitis,
2 cerebral hemorrhages and 1 uremic coma.

Our positive attitude to complete gynecological operations is now known.
The eviscerations are assessed with reservation in our department because of the
low effectiveness, especially in old women. The postoperative mortality rate
stated by *Noci et al.* (247) supports this view. In our material, we have found 7
eviscerations carried out in four gynecology departments:

Case 299/2: In this patient, an abdominal hysterectomy with both adnexae was carried out 2 years ago because of a corpus carcinoma. There is now a recurrence the size of an egg at the end of the vagina in the sigmoid region: evisceration.

Case 916/1: In this patient with an ovarian carcinoma, a recurrence occurred after an abdominal hysterectomy with both adnexae: evisceration.

Case 6/4: Ovarian carcinoma, evisceration, exitus on the 68th day after operation.

Case 390/6: Under the assumption of a collum carcinoma IV, posterior evisceration was carried out. A rectal carcinoma was found. Exitus on the 8th postoperative day.

Case 266/4: Collum carcinoma, posterior evisceration, exitus on the 21st day after operation.

Cases 453/1 and 593/1: Posterior eviscerations were carried out in preoperatively known rectal carcinoma.

Change in Surgical Geriatric Gynecology

Steinborn (290) as well as *Berle et al.* (141) are so far the only authors to have drawn attention to the qualitative changes in the analysis of the surgical material of the University Department of Gynecology, Hamburg-Eppendorf (1947–1972). They have rightly spoken of a change in surgical geriatric gynecology. They have made the following observations: (1) The increase in geriatric operations can be confirmed statistically. In the first period from 1947 to 1959, every 10th woman operated on was over 60 years old, and in the second period from 1960 to 1972 every 6th woman was over 60 years old. (2) A shift in favor of greater age is found: in the first period 22.3% of the patients operated on were over 70 years old, and in the second period 31.8%. (3) Vulvar carcinoma and kraurosis vulvae significantly increase as indication for surgery, whereas genital prolapse significantly decreases. (4) In the malignant diseases, breast carcinoma significantly increases and ovarial carcinoma decreases. (5) Simple vaginal hysterectomy without colporrhaphy as a definitive surgical procedure in genital displacement and descensus increases significantly at the cost of palliative operation such as Labhardt's or Neugebauer-Le Fort's colpocleisis. (6) Supravaginal hysterectomy with or without adnexae is hardly performed any longer. (7) Halsted mastectomy shows a significant increase, whereas simple ablatio mammae with or without checking of the axillae significantly decreases.

According to *Wittlinger* (318), the duration of the operation is the most important parameter for the intraoperative strain. In his opinion, an operation lasting less than 60 min is to be aimed for in women more than 70 years old. On the other hand, *Steinborn* (290) registered a very much longer duration of anesthesia in the years 1960–1972 compared to the years 1947–1959. Halothane-N_2O/O_2 intubation anesthesia (average duration 79.2 min) enables difficult and time-consuming operations even in elderly patients.

In agreement with the data in the literature (table 9), one can also observe a continuous increase of geriatric-gynecologic operations in the period 1960–1969 which we investigated. We also found a certain shift in favor of the higher age group in the 10-year period. We listed (1) the absolute increase in all disease groups and (2) the relative decrease in genital displacements as well as a relative rise in other disease groups associated with this. In contrast to *Steinborn* (290), we were unable to observe an absolute decline in prolapse operations. We registered with an absolute increase of all tumors, a relative increase of mammary carcinoma and a relative decrease of ovarial malignancies.

In a 10-year period, one can hardly demonstrate a marked shift between the individual surgical procedures. In agreement with *Berle et al.* (141) we observed an increase in the complete operations on genital displacement and an increase in radical mastectomy. We have already pointed out in earlier sections on the reserves still available in the optimal choice of operation.

Prevention of Geriatric-Gynecologic Diseases

Wittlinger (318) was the first to use the term 'gynecological geroprophylaxis'. In pathogenetic terms, this means the prevention of geriatric-gynecologic diseases. The best prophylaxis of these diseases is regular prevention examinations even in patients capable of bearing children. Closely related with this is an altered attitude to surgery in indicated cases in women who are in the premenopause.

Staemmler and Quaeitzsch (284) have convincingly demonstrated the justification of an extended indication for hysterectomy as a prophylactic measure in suitable cases. In recent years there has been an appreciable increase in the number of approved sterilizations. In some women in the premenopause, vaginal hysterectomy (e.g. in descensus vaginae et uteri) can be regarded as a reasonable form of sterilization.

If the removal of the adnexae in total hysterectomy hardly had any importance at the beginning of this century and earlier in 60-year-old and older women, the situation has changed in the meantime. Some authors advise against prophylactic extirpation of the adnexae in the early postmenopause on the basis of the results of former determinations. A unilateral left salpingo-oophorectomy (404) has not proved prophylactically effective against carcinoma (403).

On the contrary, we should like to speak out explicitly together with *Kofler* (401) and *Wagenbichler et al.* (405) for complete removal of the adnexae in postmenopausal women. In our department, the age limit for this is 45 years, the decision being made on an individual basis. The correctness of such an attitude is also shown by our documentation: e.g. in 42 out of 911 cases of benign ovarial tumors, at least one operation on the adnexae or the uterus had been carried out, mostly shortly before or after the menopause.

The prophylactic criteria in the indication for gynecological operations have best been described by *Kyank* (402). Intensification of cancer prevention examinations and dispensing with conservative treatment of genital displacement can be mentioned as further examples for 'gynecological geroprophylaxis' in the early postmenopause.

The remarkable proportion of 80-year-old and older women in the operation material shows that we can also speak of prevention of gynecological disease in the senium, even in the late postmenopause. We must thus look for new ways for timely registration of women in the late postmenopause. As we were able to show, a complete removal of the internal genitals is medically justified even in the late postmenopause in indicated cases.

Conclusions

6,658 operations on 60-year-old and older women were uniformly registered by one person and analyzed in the major research project of the Free University of Berlin 'Study of Statistical Systems' with the statistical programm SPSS (NORC) as well as with the information computer IBM/360-67. The significant shift within the period investigated cannot be detected in the five 5-year age groups. The average duration of treatment was 40.6 days, the preoperative preparation lasted 9.8 days and the postoperative care 30.8 days. The duration of treatment is consequently longer than that known from the literature.

We suggest the following differentiated classification for an analysis of the kinds of operation:

1	Vulvar operations
2	Vaginal operations on genital displacements
3	Abdominal or abdominovaginal operations on genital displacements
4	Vaginal operations on gynecological conditions
5	'Complete' gynecological laparotomies
6	'Incomplete' gynecological laparotomies (palliative laparotomies, exploratory laparotomies, emergency laparotomies)
7	'Complete' surgical laparotomies
8	'Incomplete' surgical laparotomies (palliative laparotomies, exploratory laparotomies, emergency laparotomies)
9	Breast operations
	In future, laparoscopy must be considered here

We formed five groups according to the kind of disease:

1	Genital displacements	1,993 women
2	Malignant tumors	3,111 women
3	Benign tumors	1,141 women
4	Other gynecological diseases	266 women
5	Other surgical diseases	147 women

The 1,993 genital displacements constituted 29.9% of the entire surgical material. A classification which has not so far been used in geriatric-gynecological literature was undertaken: (1) women with uterus, (2) women with cervical stump and (3) women with blindly ending vagina. The proportion of genital displacements (in particular descensus) decreases continuously with increasing age in the entire patient material.

Antefixation operations will soon be a thing of the past. The 22 Doléris or Kocher operations constitute merely 1.1% of all operations of genital displacements and are to be designated as 'hospital-associate'.

Vaginal hysterectomy with anterior and posterior colporrhaphy has developed to become the method of choice in the treatment of genital displacement. One can speak in descensus and prolapse treatment of a change from palliative to definitive surgical procedures. With division of the investigated period into two 5-year intervals, a lower rise is shown in descensus patients, and a marked increase in vaginal hysterectomy prolapse patients.

The number of abrasions carried out is surprisingly small in isolated vaginal colporrhaphies. Even in a semicolpocleisis, fractionated abrasion was not always carried out. Today there is only very rarely a medical indication for pessary treatment and it would be desirable if freely practising colleagues could also accept this. In vaginal or abdominal hysterectomies, the fixation of both round ligaments to the base of the vagina is necessary in order to avoid descensus or prolapse of the blind end of the vagina.

3,111 malignant tumors which were operated on constitute 46.7% of the total material and are, in contrast to the literature, the largest disease group of our operation material. Consideration of breast cancer has contributed to this. One can speak of a geriatric-oncological-gynecological triad (breast cancer, corpus carcinoma and ovarian carcinoma), and of the increasing importance of oncology in surgical geriatric gynecology. 87 vulvar carcinoma operations and 15 operations in vaginal carcinomas are not representative for the absolute frequency of these malignancies. A radiation is often preferred. Schauta and Wertheim operations are also regarded as the methods of choice in primary surgical treatment of collum carcinoma, even in geriatric patients. All other operations which are regarded as palliative (with the exception of emergency laparotomies) are to be explained either by incomplete preoperative diagnostics or inconsistency in the indication for the surgical procedure.

763 malignant tumors of the corpus uteri take first place among the operations on malignancies of the internal genitals. The only correct operation is abdominal or vaginal uterine extirpation with removal of both adnexae. The adnexae were always removed in 477 abdominal hysterectomies, but in only 71.2% of 208 vaginal hysterectomies. The same applies here to palliative operations as in collum carcinoma. With the analysis of 29 tubal carcinomas, we referred to the existing possibilities of preoperative diagnosis of this malignancy.

604 ovarian malignancies are the third most frequently operated gynecological carcinoma. Abdominal hysterectomy was carried out only 193 times (32.0%). We found an incomplete intervention in the form of a palliative operation 236 times (39.1%). Exploratory laparotomy is noticeably high with 156 cases (25.8%). The 19 emergency laparotomies (3.1%) round off the unsatisfactory picture on the surgical procedure in ovarian carcinomas. In ovarian carcinomas the time for a timely laparotomy was often passed. This underlines once more the intensification of diagnostics and preventive interventions or oophorectomy after the 45th year.

1,141 benign tumors operated on constitute 17.2% of the entire material. The evaluation of the 193 cases of uterus myomatosus contradicts the hypothesis of the postmenopausal involution of the larger myomas. Abdominal hysterectomy with adnexae has not yet sufficiently prevailed. In the 911 benign ovarian tumors, we have found abdominal hysterectomy with removal of the adnexae in 327 cases and other operations with complete removal of the remaining internal genitals in 21 cases. Misgivings concerning other surgical procedures (in our opinion incomplete) can be read in the text.

On the basis of histological examination, 56 ovarian tumors have been designated as hormonally active in our material. These were 32 granulosa cell tumors, 10 granulosa cell carcinomas, 8 thecal cell tumors and 6 Löffler-Priesel tumors. Of 21 women with bleedings before admission, an abrasion has been carried out preoperatively in only 10. We have pointed out the possible hormonal activity of some Brenner tumors and the inadequate preoperative diagnostics of hormonally active ovarian tumors.

Especially in the 266 other gynecological diseases, it is to be regretted that we decided at the beginning of the evaluation not to take small interventions into account; the importance of the precancerous gynecological conditions thus could not be adequately manifested. In 65 patients with a carcinoma in situ, 31 abdominal hysterectomies (only 3 without adnexae) and 34 vaginal hysterectomies (26 without adnexae) were carried out. A recurrent bleeding was the main indication for hysterectomy 44 times. The adnexae were removed at the same time only 20 times (17 times in 20 abdominal hysterectomies and 3 times in 24 vaginal hysterectomies). A uniform attitude to the extent of the intervention must be required if the condition is the same. This applies all the more where one must consider the possibility of a non-palpable hormonally active ovarian tumor. Here one should give preference to laparotomy so as not to have to refrain from salpingo-oophorectomy when difficulties in the surgical technique are expected.

The 282 extragenital diseases operated on mainly with gynecological diagnoses can be divided into three groups: diseases primarily operated on by gynecologists; diseases diagnosed during a laparotomy, and diseases additionally operated on. With an all-embracing interpretation of the 'extragenital diseases in surgical gynecology', a further group would have to be considered, i.e. extragenital interventions required in gynecological diseases.

In extragenital diseases, there is a subdivision into intraperitoneal extragenital and extraperitoneal (or retroperitoneal) disease pictures. In particular the retroperitoneal diseases often give rise to difficulties in differential diagnosis because of their rarity.

We suggest that the retroperitoneal diseases be subdivided gynecologically into six groups:

1	Malignant and benign, primary retroperitoneal tumors
2	Retroperitoneally located organs
3	Malignant and benign tumors of retroperitoneally located organs
4	Retroperitoneal gynecological structures
5	Retroperitoneal metastases
6	Other diseases in the retroperitoneal space

We registered 266 cases in which other gynecologic or surgical diseases were operated on apart from the underlying gynecological conditions. There are no objections in principle to operations on an additional disease. The prerequisite is the complete surgical clearing of the genital organs, i.e. treatment of underlying disease. This demand is only rarely met.

In the 6,658 cases operated on, statistical rectification of the postoperative mortality was dispensed with. The 511 postoperative deaths (7.7%) constitute a high value compared to the literature. This does not justify negative conclusions with regard to patient care in West Berlin gynecology departments. A slight dependence of the postoperative mortality on age was detected. In 60- to 64-year-old patients 5.9%, in 65- to 69-year-olds 7.8%, in 70- to 74-year-olds 8.7%, in 75- to 79-year-olds 8.9% and in 80-year-old and older patients 13.8%.

204 women (39.9%) died up to the 7th postoperative day, 113 (22.1%) died between the 8th and 14th postoperative day, 47 (9.2%) died between the 15th and 21st postoperative day, and 31 (6.1%) died between the 22nd and 28th postoperative day. A further 116 women (22.7%) died later. Of 511 women who died, 282 (55.2%) were autopsied. The proportion of 229 non-autopsied women (44.8%) is in our opinion too high. We registered a decline in autopsy frequency with increasing age of the patients. The great age of the patients who died after operations should not play any role in the decision to carry out an autopsy. The interest in an autopsy falls continuously with increasing interval between the intervention and exitus. We detected marked differences in the autopsy rate in the individual hospitals. They differ in their attitude to the importance of autopsy.

The most frequent cause of death reported was 'cardiovascular failure' with 103 cases (20.2%). However, it could be demonstrated that a 'cardiovascular failure' was almost always only the immediate cause of death and not the postoperative complication leading to exitus. The autopsy diagnosis should be broken down into underlying disease, complication leading to death, and immediate cause of death. We found the highest postoperative mortality with 13.6% in other surgical diseases. There followed malignant tumors with 12.1%, other gynecological diseases with 6.0%, benign tumors with 5.0% and genital displacements with 2.0%.

The 378 malignancy cases who died postoperatively amount to 74.0% of the entire postoperative mortality. Of importance are the low mortality rates after radical vaginal and abdominal operations in collum carcinoma (2.1 and 8.3%, respectively). Out of 604 patients with a malignant ovarian tumor, 150 (24.8%) died after the operation. The level of mortality is markedly dependent on the stage of ovarian cancer. Omission of autopsy to clarify the primary localization of the malignancy is especially regrettable in general carcinosis. The postoperative mortality is high: 51.9% in extragenital intraperitoneal malignancies and 42.1% in retroperitoneal malignancies. The overall postoperative lethality was effected only little because of the small size of these disease groups.

Breast cancer shows the lowest postoperative mortality of all malignancies with 28 deaths (2.5%). Despite of few deaths which might have been avoided, surgical treatment of breast cancer remains the method of choice, even in elderly women.

In the analysis of postoperative mortality after 57 operations on benign tumors (including 46 ovarian tumors and 8 cases of uterus myomatosus), it may not be forgotten that the surgical intervention is almost always unavoidable to clarify finally the cancer risk by means of a histological investigation even in these tumors. The 17 other gynecological diseases with lethal outcome included 4 inflammatory genital processes, 3 uterine perforations and 3 surgical corrections of urogenital fistulae. Out of 20 deaths in other surgical diseases, 15 women with a sigmoid diverticulitis take first place, followed by 4 women with appendicitis or a perityphlitic abscess.

The especially serious 40 deaths after operations of genital displacements constitute 2.0% of all descensus and prolapse operations and 7.8% of all deaths. Retrospectively, a few deaths appear to have been avoidable. With more extensive preoperative diagnostics one would probably have not carried out a surgical correction of the genital displacement. The high proportion of pulmonary embolism further points to possibilities of lowering the postoperative mortality. Despite a few regrettable deaths, the positive attitude to surgical treatment of genital displacements remains justified. Understandably, one finds the highest mortality with 51.4% in gynecological and 47.1% in surgical emergency laparotomies. Out of 249 exploratory gynecological laparotomies, 90 (26.1%) and of 88 surgical exploratory laparotomies 40 (45.5%) end lethally.

We see three possibilities of reducing the exploratory laparotomies otherwise indicated: (1) general intensification of preventive examinations in elderly women, (2) complete preoperative diagnostics and (3) application of laparoscopy.

Although we have dispensed with any statistical rectification, the postoperative mortality (7.7%) still suggests some possibilities by which it might be lowered. (1) Avoidance of non-specific and inadequate exploratory excisions, (2) timely determination of the objective palpatory finding, (3) adequate preoperative preparation, (4) complete preoperative diagnostics, (5) optimum indication for intervention, (6) in suitable cases, a laparoscopy instead of a primary laparotomy in patients who are prepared to undergo laparotomy.

The 317 women who died within the first 14 postoperative days constitute 62.0% of all patients who died. This clearly points to the main area of our efforts to lower postoperative mortality, chiefly the necessity of complex prevention and intensive treatment of postoperative complications. The necessity of an intensive postoperative care has been considered with the establishment of wards for patients recovering from anesthesia, as well as the establishment of intensive care wards. The cooperation of the gynecologists with the anesthetists is thus not only limited to the brief period of the operation but is extended to the immediate postoperative phase, and is necessary even beyond this.

The 90 cases of pulmonary embolism show that their prophylaxis before and after the intervention has not lost topicality and has remained a prime therapeutic problem in geriatric-gynecological operations. The 44 lethal bronchopneumonias prove the importance of intensive postoperative physiotherapy after geriatric operations. The organic cardiovascular diseases leading to death show the importance of the presence of multimorbidity. In principle, these should not constitute an absolute contraindication to intervention, e.g. when there is justified suspicion of a gynecological malignancy. In 72 peritonitis cases and 35 ileus cases with lethal outcome, the small number of relaparotomies is to be noted.

The advantages of the vaginal procedure compared to laparotomy are known and have also been taken into account in our patients. Processes with lethal outcome after laparotomy could not have been operated on vaginally. No recommendation in favor of the one or the other procedure can be derived from the differences in postoperative mortality in vaginal and abdominal operations.

Ultrasound examination is no more than a differential diagnostic aid in pathological findings in the true pelvis, the diagnostic advantages of laparoscopy are clear. In this connection, we point to our experience with geriatric-gynecological laparoscopies, with laparoscopic diagnostics of intestinal pathology in gynecological patients, and in a particular study on a possible lowering of the high postoperative mortality after exploratory laparotomies.

Although the number of portio stumps after supravaginal uterine amputation is not high in our operation material, we must be concerned to lower it. This means consistently carrying out a hysterectomy with adnexae. Some surgical reports indicate a certain caution of the surgeons with regard to difficult hysterectomies. We regard this as justified only in exceptionally local situations. For the experienced surgeon, hysterectomy with adnexae should not be a greater technical problem than supravaginal uterine amputation. Despite the positive attitude to complete gynecological operations, our department is cautious with regard to eviscerations in geriatric patients. In the Berlin material, we have only registered seven of these interventions.

References

General Articles

1 Kepp, R. und Staemmler, H.J.: Lehrbuch der Gynäkologie, p. 37 (Thieme, Stuttgart 1974).
2 Kern, G.: Gynäkologie. Ein kurzgefasstes Lehrbuch; 2. Aufl., p. 108 (Thieme, Stuttgart 1973).
3 Knörr, K.; Beller, F.K. und Lauritzen, C.: Lehrbuch der Gynäkologie, p. 68 (Springer, Berlin 1972).
4 Kyank, H. und Sommer, K.H.: Lehrbuch der Gynäkologie, p. 94 (VEB Georg Thieme, Leipzig 1969).
5 Lax, H.: Das endokrine System; in Stoeckel, Lehrbuch der Gynäkologie; 15. Aufl., p. 359 (Hirzel, Leipzig 1967).
6 Pschyrembel, W.: Praktische Gynäkologie; 4. Aufl., p. 536 (de Gruyter, Berlin 1968).
7 Pschyrembel, W.: Klinisches Wörterbuch; 252. Aufl., p. 1113 (de Gruyter, Berlin 1975).
8 Schrage, R.: Kompendium der Gynäkologie, p. 94 (Fischer, Stuttgart 1974).
9 Staemmler, H.J.: Fibel der gynäkologischen Endokrinologie, 2. Aufl., p. 911 (Thieme, Stuttgart 1969).

Geriatric Gynecology

10 Ahltorp, G.: Some to gynekologi. Nord. Med. 37: 12−15 (1948).
11 Alechnovich, M.V.: The importance of women's diagnostic departments for prophylaxis against genital cancer in pension age females. Vop. Onkol. 20/9: 103−106 (1974).
12 Armstrong, T.: Ginecopatias geriatricas. Vida nueva 81: 19−35 (1958).
13 Árvay, S.: A gerontológia gyneco-endocrinologiai vonatkozásai. Orv. Hétil. 109: 1625−1630 (1968).
14 Baden, W.F.: Geriatric gynecology. Postgrad. Med. 46: 241−246 (1969).
15 Barzin, P.: Pathologie gynécologique du troisième âge. Revue méd. Liège 23: 625−626 (1969).
16 Belopavlovič, M.: Pathologie gynécologique et gériatrique des malades hospitalisés à la clinique gynécologique à Novi Sad (1962−1971). Srp. Arh. celok. Lek. 100: 1041−1052 (1972).
17 Bickenbach, W.: Geriatrie aus der Sicht des Gynäkologen. Z. Geront. 1: 38−42 (1968).
18 Birnbaum, S.J.: Geriatric gynecology; in Chinn, Working with older people. A guide to practice; vol. IV: Clinical aspects of aging, pp. 149−155 (US Govt. Printing Office, Washington 1961).
19 Bláha, F.: Gerontologické problémy v současné společnosti, zvláště u žen. Čslká Gynek. 30: 409 (1965).

20 Borkowski, R.: Analiza kliniczna przypadków geriatrycznych w oddziale ginekologicznym. Wiad. lek. *20:* 2097–2102 (1967).
21 Bradford, W.Z.: The gynecologist's role in the expanding field of geriatrics. Am. J. Obstet. Gynec. *90:* 1–6 (1964).
22 Candiani, G.B.: Problemi ginecologici in geriatria. G. Geront. *25:* 115–121 (1977).
23 Cetroni, M.B.: La gerontologia ginecologica. Atti Soc. ital. Ostet. Ginec. *42:* 391–616 (1952).
24 Cetroni, M.B.: Gerontologia ginecologica. Acta geront. *3:* 13–37 (1953).
25 Cetroni, M.B.: Patologia ginecologica gerontologica. Ann. Ravasini *38:* 15 (1955).
26 Chatham, B.C.: Geriatric gynecology. J. Okla. St. med. Ass. *43:* 448–450 (1950).
27 Correa, F.: Some gynecological aspects of diseases of old age. Antiseptic *38:* 742 (1941).
28 Coyle, M.G.: Gynecological disorders in old age. Practitioner *208:* 480 (1972).
29 Davis, M.E.: Gynecology of senescence and senility; in Stieglitz, Geriatric medicine; 3rd ed., p. 555 (Lippincott, Philadelphia 1954).
30 Döring, G.: Geriatrische Gynäkologie. Mkurse ärztl. Fortbild. *27:* 508–514 (1977).
31 Douglas, C.P.: Gynaecological problems in the elderly. Practitioner *196:* 371–382 (1966).
32 Durst, F.: Ginekoloska gerijatrija. Simposion o gerontologiji. Jug. Akad. znanosti umijetnost, Zagreb 1958, pp. 249–289.
33 Echararri Ramirez, F.: Consideraciones ginecologicas en geriatria. Revta Geriat., Torreón *1:* 13–17 (1955).
34 Eddy, R.W.: Gynaecology in elderly patient. Ohio St. med. J. *44:* 1210–1212 (1948).
35 Farley, D.M. and Wolff, J.R.: Pelvic findings in women past the age of 65. J. Am. Geriat. Soc. *4:* 1–7 (1956).
36 Fernandez-Ruiz, C.: La ginecologia de la mujer vieja. Clínica Lab. *50:* 252 (1950).
37 Fernandez-Ruiz, C. e Villa, G.R.: Nuestra experiencia sobre la patologia ginecologica de la mujer vieja. Revision extadistica operatoria. Toko-ginec. práct. *22:* 293–299 (1963).
38 Folsome, C.E.; Napp, E.E., and Tanz, A.: Pelvic findings in the elderly institutionalized female patient. A gynecologic survey of six hundred eighty patients. J. Am. med. Ass. *161:* 1447–1454 (1956).
39 Foti, M.: Il trattamento anticoagulante nella geriatria ginecologica. Quad. Clin. ostet. ginec. *9:* 267–278 (1954).
40 Galloway, C.E.: Some gynecologic problems in old women. Med. Clins N. Am. *24:* 63–70 (1940).
41 Gause, R.W.: Geriatric gynecology. Trans. New Engl. obstet. gynec. Soc. *10:* 47 (1956).
42 Genell, A.S.: Gynekologens synpunkter. Nord. Med. *56:* 1057–1060 (1956).
43 Glik, I. and Soferman, N.: Gynecological survey of hospitalized elderly women. J. Am. Geriat. Soc. *19:* 61–67 (1971).
44 Glowacki, G.: Geriatric gynecology; in Reichel, Clinical aspects of aging, chapter 21, pp. 237–244 (Williams & Wilkins, Baltimore 1978).
45 Gordin, J.: Problèmes gynécologiques de la femme âgée. Revue Géront. *5:* 5 (1974).
46 Gray, M.J.: Ambulatory gynecologic services: special needs and perspectives of the aging patient. Clin. Obstet. Gynec. *20:* 183–189 (1977).
47 Grönroos, M.: Kivikoski; A.; Lehto, J., and Pulkkinen, M.O.: Postmenopausal gynecologic hospital patients. Annls Chir. Gynaec. Fenn. *57:* 168–171 (1968).
48 Gynecology of the women over sixty five. Clin. Obstet. Gynec. *10:* 443–561 (1967).

49 Hart, P.G.: Bejaarde patienten in de gynaecologische kliniek. Ned. Tijdschr. Verlosk. Gynaek. *62:* 17–30 (1962).

50 Hauser, G.A.: Altersvorgänge bei der Frau; in Schettler, Alterskrankheiten. Taschenbuch für Ärzte und Studenten, pp. 312–330 (Thieme, Stuttgart 1966).

51 Hausschild, R.: Gynäkologische Erkrankungen im Klimakterium und Senium; in Bäuschke, Doberauer und Schmidt, Leitfaden der praktischen Geriatrie (VEB Gustav Fischer, Jena 1975).

52 Heinz, M. und Hoyme, S.: Gynäkologie des Kindes- und Jugendalters (VEB Georg Thieme, Leipzig 1972).

53 Herraiz Martinez, M.; Perez Villa, I.; Rabadan Fornies, M.A. y Angulo Dominguez, J.A.: Patologia genital geriatrica. Estudio estadistico-clinico, con referencia especial a los prolapsos genitales. Revta esp. Geront. *10:* 271–280 (1975).

54 Howell, T.H. and Reade, V.: Clinical appearance of elderly women. Geriatrics *9:* 576–578 (1954).

55 Jalavisto, F. and Markonen, T.: On the assessment of biological age. II. A factorial study of aging in postmenopausal women. Annls Acad. sci. fenn. (Med.) *101:* 1–15 (1963).

56 Jalůvka, V. und Wendler, H.: Populäres über die Gynäkologie älterer und alter Frauen. Soziale Arbeit *22:* 255–256 (1973).

57 Jones, W.N.: Problems of elderly women. Sth. Surg. *10:* 203 (1941).

58 Kaiser, R. und Daume, E.: Über eine einheitliche Nomenklatur für das Klimakterium und seine Begleitsymptome. Geburtsh. Frauenheilk. *25:* 974–986 (1965).

59 Kosmak, G.W.: Gynecologic and other implications with relate to an aging female population. Am. J. Obstet. Gynec. *44:* 897–910 (1942).

60 Kosmak, G.W.: Certain aspects of gynecology as related to geriatrics. Clinics *4:* 1230–1249 (1946).

61 Kraatz, H.: Geriatrische Fragen in der Gynäkologie. Dt. GesundhWes. *16:* 1204–1209 (1961).

62 Kraatz, H.: Vorwort zu Heinz und Hoyme (52).

63 Ledermair, O.: Gynäkologische Erkrankungen im Alter. Wien. med. Wschr. *112:* 511–514 (1962).

64 Lock, F.R.: Geriatric gynecology; in Johnson, The older patient, pp. 405–421 (Holber, New York 1960).

65 Lorenzola, L.: Le affezioni ginecologiche nell'età avanzata; rilievi clinicostatistici delle affezioni ginecologiche osservati nelle donne di età superiori ai 59 anni ricoverate nella clinica L. Mangiagalli e nello Istituto Nazionale Vittorio Emanuele III dal 1928 al 1936. Annali Ostet. Ginec. *59:* 723–765 (1937).

66 Macias de Torres: La geriatria ginecologica. Revta esp. Obstet. Ginec. *18:* 134–142 (1959).

67 Manahan, C.P.: Geriatrics and gynecology. J. Philipp. med. Ass. *22:* 326 (1946).

68 Maurizio, E.: Attuali vedute di gerontologia e geriatria ginecologica. Fracastoro *48:* 577–586 (1955).

69 Mayer, A.: Bemerkungen zum Altern der Frau. Münch. med. Wschr. *76:* 219–221 (1954).

70 Mayer, A.: Bemerkungen zur gynäkologischen Gerontologie. Medizinische *50:* 2454–2459 (1959).

71 McGoogan, L.S.: Geriatric gynecology. S. Dak. J. Med. *18:* 22–25 (1965).

72 Morris, W.I.C.: Gynecological disorders in old age. Practitioner *17:* 514–520 (1953).

73 Müller, C.; Růžička, L. und Šturma, J.: Einige gynäkologische Probleme bei älteren Landfrauen. Z. Alternsforsch. *20:* 157–168 (1967).

74 Müller, C.; Růžička, L. und Šturma, J.: Die Ergebnisse prophylaktischer gynäkologischer Untersuchungen von älteren Landfrauen. Acta Univ. Carol. Med. *14:* 319–329
(1968).
75 Navratil, E. und Reiffenstuhl, G.: Geriatrische Gynäkologie; in Doberauer, Hittmair,
Nissen und Schulz, Handbuch der praktischen Geriatrie, vol. 3, pp. 524–569 (Enke,
Stuttgart 1969).
76 Ober, K.G. und Dördelmann, P.: Geriatrische Probleme in der Gynäkologie. Therapiewoche *16:* 379–385 (1966).
77 O'Sullivan, J.J.: Gynecologic problems of old age. Practitioner *165:* 141 (1950).
78 Page, E.W.: Panel on geriatric gynecology. Am. J. Obstet. Gynec. *95:* 350–365 (1966).
79 Parks, J.: Care of the postmenopausal patient. Postgrad. Med. *42:* 275–280 (1967).
80 Payne, F.L.: The gynecological care of postmenopausal patients. Delaware St. med. J.
24: 113–120 (1952).
81 Péguignot, H. et Pasquier, F.: Les problèmes gynécologiques de la femme âgée.
Concours méd. *90:* 449–458 (1968).
82 Pelegrina, I.A.: Ambulatory care of aging women: a gynecologist's point of view. Clin.
Obstet. Gynec. *20:* 177–181 (1977).
83 Pettit, W.M. de: Conditions found in the older women. Geriatrics *4:* 353–357 (1949).
84 Pettit, W.M. de; Hess, C.B., and Leibfried, J.M.: Geriatric gynecology. Surg. Clins N.
Am. *34:* 1627–1637 (1954).
85 Polatin, P. and McDonald, J.F.M.: Symposion on geriatric gynecology. Geriatrics *6:*
349–398 (1951).
86 Pratt, J.P.: Geriatric office practice. Pessaries, atrophic vaginitis, gynecologic aspects of
osteoporosis. Clin. Obstet. Gynec. *5:* 286–297 (1962).
87 Pratt, J.P.: Gynecologic problems of aging. Postgrad. Med. *37:* 213–218 (1965).
88 Quaini, P.: Gerontologia ginecologica. Studio clinico statistico sulla patologia ginecologica in pazienti oltre il 60 anno osservate nella Clinica Ostetrica e Ginecologica di
Torino (1949–1952). Acta geront. *2:* 194–200 (1952).
89 Quilez, J.: Geriatric gynecological survey. J. Newark City Hosp. *3:* 291 (1966).
90 Quinlivan, L.G.: The gynecological findings in elderly women. Geriatrics *19:* 654–657
(1964).
91 Randall, J.H.: Gynecologic problems in older women. J. Am. Geriat. Soc. *2:* 634–639
(1954).
92 Ringrose, C.A.D.: Geriatric gynecologic problems increasing. Geriatrics *33:* 389–391
(1978).
93 Rodrigues, F.V.: Ginecologia geriatrica. Relatoric oficial (Resumo). Matern. Inf. *29:*
169–173 (1970).
94 Rogers, G.: Gynecologic aspects of geriatrics. J. Okla. St. med. Ass. *41:* 321 (1948).
95 Ross, C.H.: Geriatrics and the elderly woman. J. Am. Geriat. Soc. *22:* 230–239
(1974).
96 Russell, C.S.: Gynaecology in senescence and senility; in Modern trends in geriatrics,
pp. 213–234 (Hobson, London 1956).
97 Salaber Juan, B.A.: Ginecologia geriatrica (Lopez & Edchegyen, Buenos Aires 1957);
Abstracts Revta esp. Geront. *10:* 48 (1975).
98 Sanchez Ibanez, J.M.: Ginecologia geriatrica. Revta esp. Obstet. Ginec. *27:* 475–484
(1968).
99 Scheeffey, L.C. and Lang, W.R.: The cytologic smear in gynecologic geriatric practice.
J. Am. Geriat. Soc. *1:* 348–359 (1953).
100 Schneck, P.: Zu einigen epidemiologischen und soziologischen Aspekten der ambulanten gynäkologischen Betreuung älterer Frauen. Zentbl. Gynäk. *95:* 33–40 (1973).

101 Schneck, P.: Die Frau über 60 in der gynäkologischen Ambulanz. Z. Alternsforsch. *26:* 431−433 (1973).

102 Schneider, W.: Zur Pharmakotherapie gynäkologischer Erkrankungen bei alternden und alten Frauen; in Doberauer, Scriptum geriatricum, pp. 109−116 (Gesellschaft für Geriatrie, Wien 1973).

103 Scott, R.B.: Common problems in geriatric gynecology. Am. J. Nurs. *58:* 1275−1277 (1958).

104 Sica, A. et Jorio, A. de: Considerazioni sulla patologia e ginecologia di 164 donne anziani. Rass. int. Clin. Terap. *46:* 183−201 (1966).

105 Škoda, V.; Macků, F.; Mišinger, I.; Trnka, V. a Zikmund, J.: Příčiny hospitalizace gynekologicky nemocných žen starších 60 let. Čslká Gynek. *30:* 505−508 (1965).

106 Soule, S.D.: Gynecologic disorders; in Cowdry and Steinberg, The care of the geriatric patients, chapter 8, pp. 105−111 (Mosby, St. Louis 1971).

107 Stancampiano, F.: La patologia ginecologica dell'età senile. Atti Soc. ital. Ostet. Ginec. *42:* 708−712 (1952).

108 Stark, G.: Konservative und operative Therapie gynäkologischer Erkrankungen in der Menopause. Therapiewoche *42:* 2048−2052 (1969).

109 Stieglitz, E.J.: Geriatrics gynecology. Geriatrics *6:* 347−348 (1951).

110 Stieglitz, E.J.: Foundations of geriatric medicine; in Stieglitz, Geriatric medicine; 3rd ed., pp. 3−26 (Lippincott, Philadelphia 1954).

111 Stieglitz, E.J.: Principles of geriatric medicine; in Stieglitz, Geriatric medicine; 3rd ed., pp. 27−43 (Lippincott, Philadelphia 1954).

112 Stoll, P.; Lutz, H.; Runnebaum, B. und Wittlinger, H.: Gynäkologische Erkrankungen im Klimakterium und im Senium. Ein Leitfaden für die Praxis (Deutscher Ärzte-Verlag, Köln-Lövenich 1977).

113 Traina, G. e Putignato, C.: Ginecologia della vecchiaia. Rass. Ostet. Ginec. *23:* 226−266 (1948).

114 Tropea, P.F.: Present-day aspects of gynecological gerontology. Riv. Ostet. Ginec. *15:* 421−428 (1960).

115 Turkel, W.V.; Stone, M.L., and Napp, E.E.: A geriatric gynecological survey. J. Am. Geriat. Soc. *17:* 191−195 (1969).

116 Vanrell Cruells, J.: Ginecologia geriatrica. Revta esp. Obstet. Ginec. *13:* 142 (1954).

117 Visconti, M.F. e Abbati, G.: Studio sull'incidenza della patologia geriatrica in generale e di quella ginecologica in particolare nelle ricoverate presso il Reparto Cronici degli Ospedali Riuniti di Parma nel venticinquennio 1929−53. G. Clin. med. *37:* 560−567 (1956).

118 Vojta, M.: Prevence v péči o ženy ve stáří. Čslká Gynek. *30:* 405−409 (1965).

119 Wittlinger, H.: Gynäkologische Erkrankungen in Postmenopause und Senium. Dt. Ärztebl. *70:* 2523−2326 (1973).

120 Wittlinger, H.: Geriatrie in der Gynäkologie. Klinische und morphologische Befunde bei über 60jährigen Frauen. Z. Geront. *7:* 431−440 (1974).

121 Wittlinger, H.: Geriatrie in der Gynäkologie; Habil.-Schrift Heidelberg (1973).

122 Wittlinger, H. und Dallenbach-Hellweg. G.: Blutungen in der Postmenopause und im Senium. Arch. Gynack. *211:* 459−474 (1971).

123 Würterle, A.: Alternsprobleme in Gynäkologie und Geburtshilfe. Z. Alternsforsch. *12:* 203−217 (1958).

124 Zander, J. und Baltzer, J.: Geriatrie in der Praxis aus gynäkologischer Sicht. Akt. Geront. *5:* 157−165 (1975).

125 Zerzavy, F.M.: Oncologic examinations of the institutionalized geriatric patient. Postgrad. Med. *48:* 177−179 (1970).

References   161

Surgical Geriatric Gynecology

126 Ahumada, J.C.; Nogues, A.E. y Guixa, H.L.: Patologia quirurgica ginecológica de la vejez. Día méd. *22:* 2567–2572 (1960).

127 Alicino, R. e Pietrojusti, G.: Chirurgia geriatrica ginecologica. Contributo clinico, statistico. Riv. Ostet. Ginec. prat. *43:* 649–662 (1961).

128 Alicino, R. e Zucaro, D.: Anestesia in chirurgia geriatrica ginecologica. Rass. Ostet. Ginec. *70:* 44 (1961).

129 Archilei, T.: Contributo clinico-statistico alla gerochirurgia ginecologica (premesse, aspetti e risultati della nostra esperienza). Riv. Ostet. Ginec. prat. *43:* 797–814 (1961).

130 Archilei, T. e Monti, G.B.: Anestesia in gerochirurgia ginecologica (studio clinico statistico dell'ultimo decennio). Riv. Ostet. Ginec. prat. *43:* 635–648 (1961).

131 Ardelt, W.; Dittrich, A. und Bolze, H.: Medikamentöse Thromboembolieprophylaxe in der operativen Gynäkologie der alten Frau. Geburtsh. Frauenheilk. *34:* 664–669 (1974).

132 Arenas, E. y Bettinotti, A.E.: La cirugia geriatria en la clinica ginecologica del hospital Ramos Mejia de Buenos Aires. Prensa méd. argent. *48:* 212–216 (1961).

133 Arra, J.E. et Gallucci, J.: Intervencoes ginecologicas em pacientes idosas. Anais Clin. ginec. Univ. S. Paulo *4:* 237 (1950).

134 Bagnati, E.P. y Villamayor, R.D.: La cirugia ginecológica en pacientes de mas de sessante y cinco anos. Prensa méd. argent. *44:* 973–976 (1957).

135a Balas, P.; Balaroutsos, C., and Chrysospathis, P.: Acute abdominal symptoms due to torsion of an ovarian cystadenoma in a centenarian. J. Am. Geriat. Soc. *20:* 413–415 (1972).

135b Bailo, U.; Cavezzale, C. e Finzi, C.: Considerazioni clinico-statistiche sulla chirurgia geriatrica ginecologica nel periodo 1951–1965 alla maternità provinciale di Milano. Annali Ostet. Ginec. *88:* 421–426 (1966).

136a Ballard, L.A.: Gynecologic surgery in the aging. Geriatrics *24:* 172–178 (1969).

136b Barth and Meyer; cited in Muth (241).

137 Belopavlovič, M.; Ilin, L. et Gudel, S.: Pathologie gynécologique et gériatrique des malades hospitalisés. Srp. Arh. celok. Lek. *100:* 1041–1052 (1972).

138 Belopitov, B.: Geriatrie in der operativen Gynäkologie. Vop. Pediat. Akush. Ginek., Sofia *5/5:* 51 (1961); Ber. ges. Gynäk. Geburtsh. *77:* 51 (1962).

139 Bentzen, H. and Anker, H.: Gynecological surgery in the aged. J. Oslo Cy Hosps *14:* 85–92 (1964).

140 Berger, M.; Bagovič, P.; Bolanča, M. a Puharič, I.: Ginekoloska geronto-kirurgija. Rad. med. Fak. Zagr. *18:* 199–206 (1970).

141 Berle, P.; Steinborn, H. und Thomsen, K.: Fortschritte und Wandel in der geriatrischen operativen Gynäkologie. Geburtsh. Frauenheilk. *36:* 237–246 (1976).

142 Blanchard, O. y Regueira, C.D.: La cirurgia ginecologica en geriatria. Obstet. Ginec. lat.-am. *14:* 11–20 (1956).

143 Blobel, R. und Häussler, K.: Komplikationen nach gynäkologischen Operationen bei Frauen im höheren Lebensalter. Medsche Welt *38:* 1947–1949 (1967).

144 Boguňa, I.; Palleja, J.M. y Seňor, J.C.: La cirurgia ginecológica en la anciana. Medna clín., Barcelona *30:* 111–118 (1958).

145 Bonanno, P.J.: Gynecologic problems in the elderly cardiac. J. med. Soc. New Jers. *61:* 110–112 (1964).

146 Börner, P.: Risikoklassifizierung und Risikoabwägung als Voraussetzung zur Operation von Risikopatientinnen. Geburtsh. Frauenheilk. *37:* 897–905 (1977).

147 Börner, P.; Böhme, U.; Werle, K.P. und Zimmermann, P.: Präventive Therapie allgemeiner Risiken vor gynäkologischen Operationen. Geburtsh. Frauenheilk. *38:* 1–10 (1978).

148 Bourg, R. et Piton, R.: Aspects particuliers de la chirurgie gynécologique chez les femmes âgées. Bull. Féd. Socs Gynéc. Obstét. Lang. fr. *5:* 348–354 (1953).

149 Braitenberg, H.: Über die erweiterte Indikationsstellung zu gynäkologischen Operationen an alten Patientinnen. Zentbl. Gynäk. *84:* 1569–1574 (1953).

150 Bulfoni, G.; Guidani, A. e Mannarini, G.: Consequenze della chirurgia ginecologica in pazienti anziane affette da neoplasia genitale maligna. G. Geront. *18:* 307–314 (1970).

151 Camplani, G.: Contributo clinico statistico alla ginecochirurgia gerontologica. Quad. Clin. ostet. ginec. *14:* 1227–1234 (1959).

152 Caresano, G.: La gerochirurgia nella Clinica Ostetrico-Ginecologica dell'Università di Padova dal 1950 al 1957. Atti Ostet. Ginec. *5:* 563–576 (1959).

153 Carroll, P.E. and Stoddard, F.J.: Gynecologic surgery in the aged. Obstet. Gynec., N.Y. *7:* 44–46 (1956).

154 Ceci, G.P. e Casoli, M.: La sindrome depletiva proteino-potassica nella chirurgia geriatrica ginecologica. Riv. Ostet. Ginec. *22:* 539–546 (1967).

155 Chirico, A.-M. and Rubin, A.: Medical complications of pre- and postoperative care of the elderly woman. Clin. Obstet. Gynec. *10:* 481–487 (1967).

156 Ciasca, G. e Chiaia, F.E.: La gerochirurgia nella Clinica Ostetrica e Ginecologica di Bari. Minerva ginec. *6:* 161 (1957); cited in Fioretti and Andriani (1971).

157 Crottogini, J. y Villaamil Munoz, A.: Chirurgia geriatrica en ginecologica. Scritti in onore del Prof. Tesauro (1962); cited in Verrelli (310).

158 Cséffalvay, T.; Klose, S.; Schroeter, G. und Kowasch, M.: Über Operationstoleranz und -frequenz bei gynäkologischen Eingriffen im Menopausenalter. Zentbl. Gynäk. *88:* 383–393 (1966).

159 Curiel, P. e Morresi, G.: Considerazioni clinico-statistiche in tema di chirurgia geriatrica ginecologica. Riv. Ostet. Ginec. *22:* 403–421 (1967).

160 Dalos, G.: Magy. Nöorvos. Lap. *22:* 283 (1959); cited in Horn et al. (184).

161 Danforth, W.C.: cited in Kosmak (208).

162 D'Arcangelo, G.V.; Macchione, C. e Pacilli, L.: Considerazioni in tema di anestesia peridurale segmentaria ed epidurale sacrale nella chirurgia vaginale in geriatria. Minerva ginec. *26:* 601–607 (1974).

163 Decio, R.: Considerazioni sulla chirurgia ginecologica in geriatria. G. Geront. *15:* 307–309 (1967).

164 Dieminger, H.-J.: Zur Problematik gynäkologischer Operationen im hohen Alter. Z. ärztl. Fortbild. *59:* 39–42 (1965).

165 Dlhoš, E.: Predoperačná príprava a pooperačné ošetrovanie starých žien. Čslká Gynek. *30:* 522–526 (1965).

166 Douglas, C.P.: Gynaecological surgery in the elderly. J. Obstet. Gynaec. Br. Emp. *63:* 930–931 (1956).

167 Douglas, G.W. and Studdiford, W.E.: Major gynecological surgery in the aged patient. Am. J. Obstet. Gynec. *68:* 456–465 (1954).

168 Erivancev, N.A.: Besonderheiten der Narkose und der intensiven Behandlung bei alten Frauen. Akush. Ginek. *35/9:* 56–60 (1974).

169 Eton, B.: Gynecologic surgery in elderly women. Geriatrics *28:* 119–123 (1973).

169a Felshart and Jaluvka: personal communication.

170 Ferroni, E.: La prognosi operatoria laparotomica nell'età avanzata della donna. Archo Ostet. Ginec. *20:* 311 (1933); cited in Rendina and Bellomo (265).

171 Fioretti, P. e Andriani, A.: Studio clinico sulla chirurgia geriatrica ginecologica della Clinica Ostetrica e Ginecologica di Perugia. Minerva ginec. *12:* 1092–1097 (1960).

172 Gasparri, F.; Curiel, P.; Noci, L. e Severi, S.: Indicazioni della chirurgia addominale nel vecchio. Apparato genitale femminile. Correl. Congr. Soc. Ital. Chirurgia, Firenze 1967; cited in Noci et al. (247).

173 Gause, R.W.: Geriatric gynecology at the New York Hospital. Obstet. Gynec., N.Y. *5:* 423–430 (1955).

174 Geneja, M.; Sward, J. a Wachnik, S.: Znieczulenie podczas operacji ginekologicznych u kobiet powyzej 60 roku zycia. Wiad. lek. *20:* 1521–1527 (1967).

175 Gheorghiu, N.N. und Iacob, C.: Zur gynäkologischen Chirurgie bei alten Frauen. Obstetrica Ginec., Buc. *10:* 121–125 (1963).

176 Gierdal, M. und Butters, G.: Anästhesieerfahrungen bei Altersoperationen in der Gynäkologie. Zentbl. Gynäk. *80:* 1846–1851 (1958).

177 Havlásek, L.: Morálka v operační gynecologii. Čslká Gynek. *29:* 321–325 (1964).

178 Hegyi, Z. and Radnotti, G.: Magy. Nöorvos. Lap. *22:* 277 (1959); cited in Horn et al. (184).

179 Henriquet, F.: Una classificazione del rischio operatorio per gli interventi ostetrici e ginecologici di elezione. Minerva ginec. *15:* 140–143 (1963).

180 Hilfrich, H.J.; Flaskamp, D.; Neeb, U. und Wittke, U.: Operationsrisiko und seine Beurteilung bei älteren Patientinnen. Geburts. Frauenheilk. *31:* 333–340 (1971).

181 Hilfrich, H.J.; Wittke, U.; Flaskamp, D. und Neeb, U.: Geriatrische Probleme in der operativen Gynäkologie. Dt. Ärztebl. *11:* 626–629 (1972).

182 Hochuli, E. und Bollinger, J.: Operationen bei Frauen nach der Menopause. Dt. med. Wschr. *97:* 359–363 (1972).

183 Hörmann, G.: Das Risiko bei gynäkologischen Operationen. Zentbl. Gynäk. *93:* 706 (1971).

184 Horn, B.; Szinnyai, M. und Paál, M.: Erfahrungen bei Operationen von Frauen über 60 Jahre. Zentbl. Gynäk. *85:* 1288–1295 (1963).

185 Horn, B.; Szinnyai, M., and Paál, M.: Idös nöbetegeinken végzett mütéteink tapasztalatai. Orv. Hétil. *105:* 1255–1259 (1964).

186 Horvath, U.: Idös nök. mütéti teherbírása. Magy. Nöorvos. Lap. *22:* 93–120 (1959).

187 Irmscher, A.: Operationsalter und Operationsmortalität an der Frauenklinik Karl-Marx-Stadt. Zentbl. Gynäk. *78:* 799–804 (1956).

188 Iwaszkiewicz, J.: Operacje ginekologiczne u starszych kobiet. Polski Tygod. lek. *25:* 1257–1259 (1970).

189 Jäger, G. und Pletat, D.: Die primäre Mortalität bei gynäkologischen Standardoperationen. Zentbl. Gynäk. *87:* 1393–1409 (1965).

190 Jalůvka, V.: Operative geriatrische Gynäkologie. Gynäk. Rdsch. *14:* 268–314 (1974).

191 Jalůvka, V.: Operative Behandlung des Uterus myomatosus bei 60jährigen und älteren Frauen. Geburtsh. Frauenheilk. *35:* 918–928 (1975).

192 Jalůvka, V.: Extragenitale Erkrankungen im geriatrisch-gynäkologischen Operationsgut. Zentbl. Gynäk. *98:* 275–290 (1976).

193 Jalůvka, V.: Retroperitoneale Erkrankungen und geriatrisch-gynäkologische Laparotomie. Geburtsh. Frauenheilk. *36:* 409–415 (1976).

194 Jalůvka, V.: Mammakarzinom als Bestandteil geriatrisch-gynäkologischen Operationsgutes. Z. Alternsforsch. *32:* 19–34 (1977).

195 Jalůvka, V.: Grössere gynäkologische Operationen bei 80jährigen und älteren Frauen. Arch. Gynaek. *122:* 73–93 (1977).

196 Jalůvka, V.: Probelaparotomie im geriatrisch-gynäkologischen Operationsgut. Geburtsh. Frauenheilk. *37:* 317–321 (1977).

Surgical Geriatric Gynecology 164

197 Jalůvka, V.: Hysterektomie bei geriatrischen Patientinnen. Fortschr. Med. *92:* 1429–1432 (1977).
198 Jalůvka, V. und Felshart, K.-J.: Primäre Pathologie des Sigma und des Rektum bei geriatrisch-gynäkologischer Laparotomie. Geburtsh. Frauenheilk. *35:* 10–20 (1975).
199 Jalůvka, V.; Langbein, L. und Herold, G.: Frühmortalität im geriatrisch-gynäkologischen Operationsgut. Zentbl. Gynäk. *99:* 407–418 (1977).
200 Jalůvka, V.; Lübke, F. und Zielske, F.: Geriatrisch-gynäkologische Laparoskopie (personal communication).
201 Junge, W.-D.; Daub, I.; Stark, K.H. und Benad, G.: Blutanalysen in der operativen geriatrischen Gynäkologie. Zentbl. Gynäk. *98:* 1430–1433 (1976).
202 Károlyi, T.: Operačný profil výše 60 ročných žien. Čslká Gynek. *26:* 684–688 (1961).
203 Kenmotsu, O., et al.: Anesthetic management in surgery of a giant ovarian tumor in an aged patient. Jap. J. Anaesth. *20:* 357–362 (1971).
204 Kindermann, G.: Operative Probleme der Gynäkologie bei den älteren Frauen. Klinikarzt *6:* 136–143 (1977).
205 Klejna, F.; Macků, F. a Trnka, V.: Anesteziologické problémy při operacích starých žen. Čslká Gynek. *30:* 526–529 (1965).
206 Kolářová, O. und Staníček, J.: Die gegenwärtigen Ergebnisse und weiteren Perspektiven der operativen Heilung älterer Frauen in der Gynäkologie. Scr. med. Fac. Med. Brno *39:* 67–72 (1966).
207 Kolos, Á. és Ferkó, S.: Tapasztalataink és eredményeink a 60 év feletti betegeken végzett nagyobb nögyógyászati mütétek kapcsán. Magy. Nöorvos. Lap. *37:* 403–406 (1974).
208 Kosmak, G.W.: Gynecologic and other implications which relate to an aging female population. Am. J. Obstet. Gynec. *44:* 897–910 (1942).
209 Krango, D.; Lazarov, A. i Jurukovski, J.: Operativno lekuvanje na stari ženi, Godišen Zb. med. Fak. Skopje *13:* 249–255 (1966).
210 Krupa, B.; Lipski, J. i Wojdala, Z.: Operacje ginekologiczne po 65 roku zycia. Ginek. pol. *39:* 91–94 (1968).
211 Kvíz, D.: V čem je možno spatřovat příčiny poklesu křivky gynekologické operační mortality? Čslká Gynek. *24:* 404–406 (1964).
212 Lash, A.F.: Surgical geriatric gynecology. Am. J. Obstet. Gynec. *53:* 766–775 (1947).
213 Lash, A.F.: Gynecologic surgery in the elderly women. Geriatrics *3:* 67–71 (1948).
214 Lash, A.F.: Current concepts of surgical geriatric gynecology. Int. Surg. *60:* 71–74 (1975).
215 Lazar, M.R. and Snider, E.U.: New hemostatic agent for geriatric gynecology. Obstet. Gynec., N.Y. *27:* 341–346 (1966).
216 Lefèvre: Forh. Nord. For. Obst. Gyn. Congress, Oslo 1956, p. 140; cited in Bentzen and Anker (139).
217 Leinzinger, E.: Alterschirurgie in der Gynäkologie. Neue Rundschau für Prophylaxe, Diagnostik und Therapie 1963, Heft 3/4; zitiert in Wittlinger (318).
218 Levinson, V.B. and Potanova, O.N.: Features peculiar to anesthesia during gynecological operations in old patients. Akush. Ginek. *40/6:* 77–80 (1964).
219 Levy, J. et Melchior, J.: Chirurgie gynécologique de la femme âgée. Revue fr. Gynéc. Obstét. *67:* 147–152 (1972).
220 Lewis, A.C.W.: Major gynecological surgery in the elderly. A review of 305 patients. J. int. Fed. Gynaec. Obstet., Napoli *6:* 244–258 (1968).
221 Liccione, W.T.: Am. J. Surg. *29:* 236 (1935); cited by Lash (212).
222 Lopatecki, T.; Dusza, M. a Zurawik, Z.: Operacje ginekologiczne po 60 roku zycia. Wiad. lek. *22:* 1471–1472 (1969).

223 Loskant, G.: Das Risiko der gynäkologischen Alterschirurgie. Saarl. Ärztebl. 8: Heft 8, pp. 1–8 (1968).
224 Loskant, G.: Gynäkologische Operationen an alten Patienten. Geburtsh. Frauenheilk. 28: 492–497 (1968).
225 Lucisano, F.: Aspetti particolari della chirurgia ginecologica nelle pazienti di età avanzata (Rilievi clinico-statistici sulla casistica dell'ultimo decennio). Clinica ostet. ginec. 62: 1–29 (1960).
226 Macků, R. a Kubečka, A.: Naše zkušenosti s operativní léčbou u starých žen. Čslká Gynek. 27: 539–543 (1962).
227 Mai, J.: Ergebnisse gynäkologischer Operationen bei Patientinnen über 60 Jahre. Zentbl. Gynäk. 94: 33–39 (1972).
228 Malato, M. e Arienzo, R.: Rilievi in tema di gerontochirurgia ginecologica. Archo Ostet. Ginec. 75: 235–244 (1970).
229 Manahan, C.P.: Geriatrics and gynecology; role of surgery in the aged. J. Philipp. med. Ass. 22: 326 (1946).
230 Mattingly, R.F.: Surgery in the aging female. Clin. Obstet. Gynec. 7: 573–602 (1964).
231 Maurizio, E. e Pescetto, G.: Gli interventi chirurgici in donne oltre i 60 anni presso la Clinica Ostetrica e Ginecologica di Genova nel quadriennio 1951–1954. Minerva med. 47: 1524–1526 (1956).
232 Mauzey, A.J. and Kaknes, G.B.: Pelvic surgery in the elderly psychiatric woman. J. Am. Geriat. Soc. 1: 272–279 (1953).
233 Mayer, H.G.K.: Leitungsanästhesie in der geriatrischen Gynäkologie. Geburtsh. Frauenheilk. 34: 203–206 (1974).
234 McKeithen, W.S., Jr.: Major gynecologic surgery in the elderly female 65 years of age and older. Am. J. Obstet. Gynec. 123: 59–65 (1975).
235 Mengaldo, R.: Nostro contributo clinico in gerochirurgia ginecologica. Minerva ginec. 11: 112–115 (1962).
236 Michalangeli, F., et al.: Methods and indications for low peridural analgesia in the aged. Report of 300 cases. Ann. Anesth. fr. 18: 524–534 (1977).
237 Mikulicz-Radecki, F. von: Das Alter der wegen einer gynäkologischen Erkrankung bei uns operierten Frauen. Zentbl. Gynäk. 78: 1241–1250 (1956).
238 Mirkov, K. and Atanasov, D.: Characteristics of gynecologic operations in aged women. Akush. Ginec., Sofia 9: 135–142 (1970).
239 Mosler, W.: Das Operationsrisiko bei alten Frauen. Zentbl. Gynäk. 89: 1106–1111 (1967).
240 Moustamindy, N.: Aspects actuels de la chirurgie gynécologique du 3e âge à la clinique gynécologique de Lyon. Bull. Féd. Socs Gynéc. Obstét. Lang. fr. 23: 183–188 (1971).
241 Muth, H.: Zur gynäkologischen Alterschirurgie unter besonderer Berücksichtigung der vaginalen Operationsmethoden. Geburtsh. Frauenheilk. 31: 1202–1214 (1971).
242 Mussey, R.T.: cited in Kosmak (208).
243 Myasischev, G.F.: Laparotomy in gynecological patients of advanced age. Akush. Ginek. 35/4: 91–94 (1959).
244 Navratil, E.: Indikation, Gefahren und Ergebnisse gynäkologischer Operationen bei alten Frauen; in Doberauer, Geriatrie und Fortbildung, pp. 169–177 (Burgland Druckerei, Wien 1960).
245 Niesert, W. und Seidenschnur, G.: Operationen an alten Frauen. Z. Geburtsh. Gynäk. 150: 249–263 (1958).
246 Nobile, T.; Balocco, G. e Noca, R.: La nostra esperienza in chirurgia gerontologica. Archo Sci. med. 126: 340–344 (1965).

247 Noci, L.; Curiel, P. e Laurentiis, G. de: Le eviscerazioni pelviche in età geriatrica. Riv. Ostet. Ginec. *23:* 766–776 (1968).

248 Notelowicz, M.: Tolerance of elderly patients to major gynaecological surgery. S. Afr. med. J. *46:* 1618–1621 (1972).

249 Novotný, A. a Dvořák, V.: Vliv stáří na tromboembolickou nemoc v gynekologii. Čslká Gynek. *30:* 544–548 (1968).

250 O'Leary, J.A. and Symmonds, R.E.: Radical pelvic operations in the geriatric patient. A 15-year review of 133 cases. Obstet. Gynec., N.Y. *28:* 745–753 (1966).

251 Paldi, E.; Hoch, Z.; Pascal, B. et Peretz, A.: Opérations gynécologiques dans l'âge gériatrique. Revue fr. Gynéc. Obstét. *67:* 159–161 (1972).

252 Paldi, E.; Peretz, A., and Pascal, B.: Gynecologic surgery in geriatric patients. Geriatrics *21:* 131–136 (1966).

253 Palik, F.: Magy. Nöorvos. Lap. *22:* 278 (1959); cited in Horn et al. (184).

254 Palmrich, A.H.: Mortalität und Operabilität in der gynäkologischen Geriatrie; in Doberauer, Medizinische und soziale Altersprobleme, pp. 277–285 (Verlag Gesellschaft zur Förderung wissenschaftlicher Forschung, Wien 1958).

255 Pernecker, E.: Betäubungsverfahren bei gynäkologischen Eingriffen im höheren Lebensalter an der Universitätsfrauenklinik Berlin von 1950–1961; Inaug. Diss. Berlin (1965).

256 Piechowiak, Z.; Mazurova, A. a Krakowska, B.: Przygotowania do operacji ginekologicznych chorych w wieku starszym. Ginek. pol. *45:* 575–580 (1974).

257 Pierson, R.L.; Figge, P.K., and Buchsbaum, H.J.: Surgery for gynecologic malignancy in the aged. Obstet. Gynec., N.Y. *46:* 523–527 (1975).

258 Piton, R.V.: La chirurgie gynécologique chez les femmes agées. Bull. Soc. r. belge Gynéc. Obstét. *28:* 267–274 (1958).

259 Pócsy, G. és Nemecskay, T.: Magy. Nöorvos. Lap. *22:* 277 (1959); cited in Horn et al. (184).

260 Polito, P.M.; Gentile, D.; Stanca, A. e Pelusi, G.: Morbidità in chirurgia geriatrica ginecologica. Riv. ital. Ginec. *51:* 834–844 (1967).

261 Pratt, J.H.: Gynecologic surgery in the geriatric patients. J. Ark. med. Soc. *52:* 173 (1956).

262 Quaini, P. e Colla, G.: Indicazioni e contraindicazioni della terapìa chirurgica nella gerontologica ginecologica. Acta geront. *5:* 305–338 (1955).

263 Randow, H. und Riess, D.: Besonderheiten grosser gynäkologischer Operationen bei alten Frauen. Dt. GesundhWes. *21:* 1459–1464 (1966).

264 Reichelt, O.: Gynäkologische Operationen bei alten Leuten. Vor- und Nachbehandlung. Wien. med. Wschr. *87:* 119–121 (1937).

265 Rendina, G.M. e Bellomo, P.: Chirurgia geriatrica ginecologica. Minerva ginec. *17:* 923–927 (1965).

266 Rieppi, G.; Cargnello, U. e Nadali, L.: Problemi clinico-anestesiologici/gerochirurgia ginecologica. Friuli med. *20:* 803–838 (1965).

267 Rigó, J. und Zubek, L.: Erfahrungen bezüglich der Anamnesen und Operationen von gynäkologischen Patienten über 60 Jahre. Zentbl. Gynäk. *92:* 1718–1724 (1970).

268 Rio, F.: In tema di gerontochirurgia. Clinica ostet. ginec. *71:* 112–119 (1969).

269 Rolandi, L. e Corti, A.: Sulla chirurgia geriatrica ginecologica praticata nell'Ospedale Maggiore di Milano nel decennio 1951–1960. Clinica ginec. *4:* 356 (1961); cited in Bailo et al. (135b).

270 Rupprecht, A. und Stange, H.-H.: Über die operative Behandlung der über 70jährigen Frauen an der Univ. Frauenklinik Kiel in den Jahren 1929 bis 1958. Zentbl. Gynäk. *82:* 1089–1095 (1960).

271 Rusch, H.P.: 1000 gynäkologische Operationen im Greisenalter. Geburtsh. Frauen-heilk. *6:* 211–217 (1944).
272 Sakamoto, S., et al.: Aging and gynecologic operations. Sanfujinha Jissai *20:* 330 (1971).
273 Schiller, W.: Gynäkologische Operationen bei Greisinnen. Medsche Welt *20:* 1152–1156 (1962).
274 Schilling, H. und Schneck, P.: Gynäkologische Operationen bei alten Patientinnen. Dt. GesundhWes. *24:* 2263–2269 (1969).
275 Schulze, H.: Zur Frage der Narkosebelastung bei den Todesfällen in der operativen Frauenheilkunde und Geburtshilfe. Zentbl. Gynäk. *89:* 1633–1639 (1967).
276 Schürmann, K.: Ein Beitrag zur Problematik der operativen gynäkologischen Therapie bei Patientinnen im Greisenalter. Zentbl. Gynäk. *87:* 745–755 (1965).
277 Sieroszewski, J.; Piechowiak, Z.; Mazurova, A. a Krakowska, B.: Operacje ginekologiczne i przebieg pooperacyjny u chorych po 60. roku zycia. Ginek. pol. *45:* 451–458 (1974).
278 Siliquini, P.N.: Considerazioni clinico statistiche di 220 interventi in donne oltre i 60 anni di età. Atti Soc. ital. Ostet. Ginec. *42:* 703–705 (1952).
279 Siliquini, P.N. e Petterino, E.: Analisi comparativa di dati biologici e clinici del de-corso post operatorio in chirurgia ginecologica geriatrica. G. Geront. *17:* 1159–1187 (1969).
280 Sirtori, C.M.: Chirurgia geriatrica ginecologica. (Rilievi clinico-statistici). Quad. Clin. ostet. ginec. *14:* 1186–1200 (1959).
281 Skiftis, T.; Piskazeck, K. und Schmidt, L.: Über die operative Behandlung von über 60 Jahre alten Patientinnen. Zentbl. Gynäk. *85:* 1725–1730 (1963).
282 Smith, L.R. and Pratt, J.H.: Vaginal hysterectomy in the geriatric patient. Obstet. Gynec., N.Y. *13:* 84–91 (1959).
283 Soferman, N.; Glick, I. et Horenstein, I.: Contribution à la chirurgie gériatrique. Revue fr. Gynéc. Obstét. *67:* 153–155 (1972).
284 Staemmler, H.J. und Quaeitzsch, V.: Über die Problematik der präoperativen Hysterek-tomie. Geburtsh. Frauenheilk. *32:* 89–96 (1972).
285 Stafeeva, E.N., et al.: Peridural anaesthesia in gynecological patients of advanced age. Sov. Med. *4:* 109–111 (1977).
286 Stanca, A.; Dalla Pria, S.; Piccolomini, A. e Pelusi, G.: La chirurgia geriatrica nella Clinica Ostetrica e Ginecologica di Siena. Riv. ital. Ginec. *51:* 750–765 (1967).
287 Starostina, T.A.: Gynecological operations in aged and senile women. Akush. Ginek. *39/2:* 38–44 (1963).
288 Starostina, T.A.: Gynecological operations in aged and senile women suffering from cardiovascular diseases. Akush. Ginek. *42/4:* 14–17 (1966).
289 Štefánik, S.: Rizikooperacie u starých žien. Čslká Gynek. *30:* 529–534 (1965).
290 Steinborn, H.: Fortschritte und Wandel in der geriatrischen operativen Gynäkologie; Inaug. Diss. Hamburg (1975).
291 Stožický, V. a Vácha, K.: Kontraindikace operací u starých žen. 'Komplikace a kontraindikace operační léčby'. Čsl. věd. konf. porod. a gynek. spol. J.E. Purkyně, Brno 1967, pp. 179–188.
292 Strobel, E.: Ergebnisse nach 6,251 grösseren gynäkologischen Operationen zwischen 1950 und 1969 unter besonderer Berücksichtigung der Embolieletalität. Zentbl. Gynäk. *92:* 577–584 (1970).
293 Suonoja, L.; Ylikorkala, O., and Järvinen, P.A.: Gynecologic surgery in elderly patients. Annls Chir. Gynaec. Fenn. *64:* 388–393 (1975).
294 Szarka, S.: Magy. Nöorvos. Lap., p. 154 (1941); cited in Horn et al. (184).
295 Szendi, B.: Magy. Nöorvos. Lap. *22:* 281 (1959); cited in Horn et al. (184).

296 Szendi, B. und Lakatos, I.: Beziehungen zwischen Gynäkologie und Geriatrie unter der Landbevölkerung. Z. ärztl. Fortbild. *53:* 1208–1214 (1959).
297 Tancer, M.L. and Matseoane, S.L.: Gynecologic surgery in patients over 65. Geriatrics *21:* June 189–196 (1966).
298 Tancinco-Yambao, G. and Lopez, A.: Aging women as surgical patients. Philipp. J. Surg. *8:* 145–149 (1953).
299 Te Linde, R.: cited in Kosmak (208).
300 Terzi, I.; Lucci, U. e Pavetto, P.F.: Ginecologia operativa gerontologica. Studio clinico statistico. G. Geront. *14:* 277–288 (1966).
301 Torsello, R. e Palazzetti, P.: Ricerche sul volume totale del sangue e crasi ematica in gerontologia ginecologica. Atti Ostet. Ginec. *3:* 109–113 (1959).
302 Trebicka, B.: Operacje ginekologiczne u kobiet w podeszlym wieku. Przegl. lek. *11:* 169–173 (1955).
303 Trnka, V.: Operační výsledky a risiko gynekologických operací u žen starších 60 let. Čslká Gynek. *22:* 177–183 (1957).
304 Uhlmann: Diskussion zu Rupprecht und Stange. Zentbl. Gynäk. *82:* 802 (1960).
305 Uzel, R. a Kolářová, O.: K otázce operační léčby velmi starých žen. Čas. Lék. česk. *108:* 467–469 (1969).
306 Vácha, K.: Operace u žen ve stáří. Čslká Gynek. *30:* 509–521 (1965).
307 Vácha, K. a Stožický, V.: Operace starých žen. Čslká Gynek. *29:* 380–383 (1964).
308 Valle, G.: L'operabilità ginecologica nelle vecchie. Minerva ginec. *7:* 599–602 (1955).
309 Velikay, L.: Die Operationsmortalität an der II. Universitäts-Frauenklinik Wien. Zentbl. Gynäk. *77:* 577–583 (1955).
310 Verrelli, D.: Aspetti della chirurgia geriatrica ginecologica. Quad. Clin. ostet. ginec. *22:* 95–109 (1967).
311 Verrelli, D.: Rilievi clinici sugli interrenti ginecologici nell'età geriatrice. Quad. Clin. ostet. ginec. *22:* 110–120 (1967).
312 Weed, J.C. and Mighell, J.R.: Major gynecologic operations in the patient over 50 years of age. Am. J. Obstet. Gynec. *59:* 305–310 (1950).
313 Wendl, H.K.: Anaesthesie im Greisenalter. Arch. Gynaek. *195:* 295–298 (1961).
314 Widholm, O.; Kivalo, I., and Nieminen, U.: Gynaecological operations on geriatric patients. Annls Chir. Gynaec. Fenn. *54:* 91–100 (1965).
315 Wille, P.; Randow, H. und Riess, D.: Vegetatives System und postoperative Thrombo-Embolie bei älteren gynäkologischen Patienten. Geburtsh. Frauenheilk. *27:* 500–508 (1967).
316 Wittig, R.: Über Probleme bei der präoperativen Behandlung alter Patienten. Zentbl. Gynäk. *97:* 1394–1397 (1975).
317 Wittlinger, H.: Gynäkologische Operationen bei über 60jährigen Patientinnen. Therapiewoche *22:* 2063–2067 (1972).
318 Wittlinger, H.: Geriatrie in der Gynäkologie. Klinische und morphologische Befunde bei über 60jährigen Frauen. Z. Geront. *7:* 431–440 (1974).
319 Woraschk, H.J.: Zum postoperativen Verlauf bei Greisinnen. Dt. GesundhWes. *15:* 600–602 (1960).
320 Zelkind, G.B. und Djagilev, I.I.: Einige Besonderheiten der postoperativen Periode in der geriatrischen Gynäkologie. Sov. Med. *8:* 151 (1974).
321 Zeman, F.D. and Davids, A.M.: Gynecologic surgery in the elderly with special reference to risk and results. Am. J. Obstet. Gynec. *56:* 440–456 (1948).
322 Zielske, F. und Jalůvka, V.: Die Bedeutung der gynäkologischen Laparoskopie bei Erkrankungen des Colon sigmoideum im Alter. Fortschr. Med. *96:* 1129–1132 (1978).

Geriatric Problems of Hormonally Active Ovarian Tumors

323 Aiman, J.; Nalick, R.H.; Jacobs, A.; Porter, J.C.; Edman, C.D.; Vellios, F., and MacDonald, P.C.: The origin of androgen and estrogen in a virilized postmenopausal woman with bilateral benign cystic teratomas. Obstet. Gynec., N.Y. *49:* 659–704 (1977).

324 Assen, F.J.J. van: Een patients met een zer kleine ovariumtumor. Ned. Tijdschr. Geneesk. *109:* 2063–1064 (1965).

325 Behrens, H.: Genitalblutungen als Folge kleinster, nicht palpabler Ovarialtumoren. Z. Geburtsh. Gynäk. *139:* 182–197 (1953).

326 Behrens, H.: Hormonuntersuchungen bei Frauen mit Ovarialtumoren in der Menopause. Arch. Gynaek. *193:* 270–278 (1959).

327 Bhargava, V.L.: Hormonal activity of 'non-functioning' ovarian tumor. Aust. N.Z. J. Obstet. Gynec. *9:* 108–115 (1969).

328 Bilde, T.: Ovarian stromal hyperplasia associated with hyperoestrogenism in a postmenopausal woman. Acta obstet. gynec. scand. *46:* 429–434 (1967).

329 Brody, S.: Ovarian cysts with hormonal activity. Int. Surg. *46:* 244–245 (1966).

330 Brux, J. et Dorangeon, P.: Tumeur ovarienne à type de thécome contenant des cellules de Leydig avec syndrome d'hyperfolliculinie chez une femme ménopausée. Bull. Féd. Socs Gynéc. Obstét. Lang. fr. *11:* 104–111 (1959).

331 Christensen, I. and Toft, G.: Feminizing luteoma of the ovary. Acta obstet. gynec. scand. *32:* 389–398 (1953).

332 Cianfrani, T.: A minute granulosa cell tumor, with vaginal bleeding. Ann. Surg. *124:* 118–122 (1946).

333 Delattre, A.; Gaudefroy, M. et Camus, H.: Tumeur de la granulosa diagnostiquée par la cytologie vaginale. J. Sciences méd. Lille *72:* 272–274 (1954).

334 Detlefsen, M.: Postklimakterische Blutungen durch follikelhormonbildende Ovarialtumoren (Oestroblastome). Eine nicht seltene, aber in der Praxis wenig bekannte und oft übersehene Blutungsursache. Dt. GesundhWes. *12:* 425–429 (1957).

335 Dhom, G.: Zur Topographie und Histogenese kleinster Brennertumoren. Arch. Gynaek. *184:* 32–39 (1953).

336 Edwards, R.L.; Nicholson, H.O.; Zoidis, T.; Butt, W.R., and Taylor, C.W.: Endocrine studies in post-menopausal women with ovarian tumours. J. Obstet. Gynaec. Br. Commonw. *78:* 467–477 (1971).

337 Erb, M.: Diagnostisches und therapeutisches Vorgehen bei kleinen Ovarialtumoren. Praxis *65:* 167–171 (1976).

338 Eriksen, H.C.: Postklimakterial metrorrhagi forarsaget af granulosacelletumorer. Nord. Med. *65:* 73–75 (1961).

339 Esin, G.S.: Zytologische Befunde bei hormonal wirksamen Ovarialtumoren in der Menopause. Zentbl. Gynäk. *90:* 1305–1308 (1968).

340 Fathalla, M.F.: The occurrence of granulosa and theca tumours in clinically normal ovaries. J. Obstet. Gynaec. Br. Commonw. *74:* 279–282 (1967).

341 Fienberg, R.: Ovarian estrogenic tumors and diffuse estrogenic thecomatosis in postmenopausal colporrhagia. Am. J. Obstet. Gynec. *76:* 851–860 (1958).

342 Fienberg, R.: The stromal theca cell and postmenopausal endometrial adenocarcinoma. Cancer *24:* 32–38 (1969).

343 Flickinger, G.L.; Murawec, T., and Touchstone, J.C.: Free and conjugated estrogens of an ovarian cystadenoma and granulosa cell tumor. J. clin. Endocr. Metab. *25:* 1231–1236 (1965).

344 Francis, M.M.: Granulosa cell tumor of the ovary at the age of 85 years. J. Obstet. Gynaec. Br. Emp. *64:* 274–275 (1957).

345 Gaudefroy, M.: Value of vaginal cytology. J. Sciences méd. Lille *82:* 495–497 (1964).
346 Gennaro, D. de: Tumore di Krukenberg funzionante in menopausa. Minerva ginec. *14:* 225–229 (1962).
347 Genton, C.: Ein Sertoli-Leydig-Zelltumor als Zufallsbefund bei einer 72jährigen Patientin. Zentbl. Gynäk. *100:* 154–156 (1978).
348 Giron Blanc, J.J.: Un caso de tumor funcionante de ovario en la menopausia. Revta esp. Obstet. Ginec. *29:* 264–268 (1961).
349 Groot-Wassink, K.; Stahl, F.; Wiern, L.; Fischer, M.; Ittrich, G.; Richter, J.; Herrmann, V. und Dietz, K.: Lokalisation eines kleinen androgenaktiven Ovarialtumors durch Katheterisierung der Venen femoralis und selektive Venenblutabnahme mit Testosteronbestimmung im Plasma. Zentbl. Gynäk. *97:* 1304–1309 (1975).
350 Harris, H.R.: Granulosa cell tumor of the ovary. Report of a case in a woman aged 82 years. J. Obstet. Gynaec. Br. Emp. *64:* 272–273 (1957).
351 Hermann, E.: Granulosa- und Thekazelltumoren als Ursache rezidivierender glandulär-cystischer Hyperplasien der Corpusschleimhaut. Medsche Klin. *53:* 1337–1339 (1958).
352 Hermann, E.: Granulosa- bzw. Thekazelltumoren, ihre Genese und ihre Beziehung zum Adenokarzinom des Corpus uteri. Z. Geburtsh. Gynäk. *144:* 154–171 (1955).
353 Herold, J. and Papež, L.: Evaluation of the hormonal activity of ovarian carcinoma in comparing vaginal smears with mammography. Acta cytol. *11:* 439–443 (1967).
354 Hollstein: Ein seltener hormonbildender Ovarialtumor. Zentbl. Gynäk. *72:* 1609 (1950).
355 Huber, H.: Thekazelltumor als Blutungsursache in der Menopause. Zentbl. Gynäk. *61:* 14–17 (1937).
356 Jalůvka, V. und Felshart, K.J.: Granulosazelltumor bei Greisinnen. Zentbl. Gynäk. *93:* 348–352 (1971).
357 Jalůvka, V. und Kratzsch, E.: Granulosazell- und Brennertumor bei Patientin mit Adenocarcinoma corporis uteri. Zentbl. Gynäk. *95:* 603–608 (1973).
358 Jalůvka, V. und Kratzsch, E.: Zur Hormonaktivität einiger Brennertumoren (personal communication).
359 Jones, G.S. und Woodruff, J.D.: Granulosa-cell-tumor diagnosis by urinary-estrogen assay. Obstet. Gynec., N.Y. *22:* 214–218 (1963).
360 Kecskes, L.: Isolation of estrone from the urine of a patient with ovarian cancer. Orv. Hétil. *105:* 152–156 (1969).
361 Kecskes, L.; Mutschler, F. und Kobor, J.: Östrogenbestimmungen im Gewebe bei Tumoren der Ovarien. Zentbl. Gynäk. *85:* 325–328 (1963).
362 Keller, B.; Levy, G. et Philippe, E.: Hyperfolliculinie postménopausique par tumeurs sécrétantes de l'ovaire: à propos de deux cas. Bull. Féd. Socs Gynéc. Obstét. Lang. fr. *16:* 615–617 (1964).
363 Klöppner, K.: Thekazellgeschwulst mit Dauerblutungen in der Menopause und Fibromyom des Uterus bei 69jähriger Patientin mit Zeichen von Verjüngung. Medizinische *47:* 576–577 (1953).
364 König, F.E.: Granulosa- und Thekazelltumoren und Scheidenabstrich. Gynaecologia *135:* 225–228 (1953).
365 Kyank, H.: Ein besonders kleiner Granulosazelltumor als Ursache einer rezidivierenden glandulären Hyperplasie nach Röntgenkastration. Zentbl. Gynäk. *71:* 250–254 (1949).
366 Lahm, W.: Zur Frage der postklimakterischen Blutungen bei Ovarialkarzinom und Adenom der Matrone. Zentbl. Gynäk. *51:* 2743–2746 (1927).
367 Le Lièvre, H. et Isidor, P.: Métrorragies post-ménopausiques dues à une tumeur complexe de l'ovarie hormone-sécrétante. Gynéc. Obstét. *54:* 441–451 (1955).
368 MacDonald, P.C.; Grodin, J.M.; Edman, C.D.; Vellios, F., and Siiteri, P.K.: Origin of

estrogen in a postmenopausal woman with a nonendocrine tumor of the ovary and endometrial hyperplasia. Obstet. Gynec., N.Y. *47:* 644–650 (1976).

369 MacDonald, T.W.; Malkasian, G.D., and Gaffey, T.A.: Endometrial cancer associated with feminizing ovarian tumor and polycystic ovarian disease. Obstet. Gynec., N.Y. *49:* 654–658 (1977).

370 Massobrio, E.: Early diagnosis of tumors of the endocrine system. Cancer *16:* 280–297 (1963).

371 Maxwell, D.M.W.: Granulosa cell tumor producing symptoms four years following radium menopause. J. Obstet. Gynaec. Br. Emp. *63:* 232–233 (1956).

372 Mizejewski, G.J.; Beierwaltes, W.H., and Quinones, J.: Uptake of radioiodinated human chorionic gonadotropic hormone by ovarian carcinoma. J. nucl. Med. *13:* 101–106 (1971).

373 Monrozies, M. et Planel, H.: Métrorragies post-ménopausiques par tumeur de la granulosa. Bull. Féd. Socs Gynéc. Obstét. Lang. fr. *11:* 562–566 (1959).

374 Moretti, G.; Broustet, A.; Beylot, J.; Amouretti, M. et Delaunay, M.: Menstruation paradoxale et ascite intarissable par tumeur de la 'granulosa' dans la post-ménopause. Intérêt de l'étude cytogénétique du liquide d'ascite. Sem. Hôp. Paris *49:* 645–648 (1973).

375 Müllerheim, R.: Ovarialtumoren bei Greisinnen mit Hypertrophie der Mammae und des Uterus und mit uterinen Blutungen. Zentbl. Gynäk. *52:* 689–693 (1928).

376 Nevinny-Stickel, J.: Thekazelltumor und Korpuskarzinom bei einer 75jährigen Frau. Zentbl. Gynäk. *78:* 1640–1644 (1956).

377 Ozieblo, L.; Roszkowski, I.; Kasperlik-Zaluska, A.; Szamborski, J.; Teter, J.; Guzel, L., and Baranowska, B.: Hormonalnie czynny guz jajnika jako przyczyna wirylizacji po menopauzie. Endokr. pol. *25:* 377–382 (1974).

378 Patterson, J.H.; McCullagh, H., and Mck, W.: A case of thecacell tumour of the ovary in a women aged 92 years. J. Obstet. Gynaec. Br. Emp. *43:* 1186–1190 (1936).

379 Procopé, B.J.: Studies on the urinary excretion, biological effects and origin of oestrogens in post-menopausal women. Acta endocr., Copenh. *60:* 5 (1969).

380 Rauramo, L.; Grönroos, M., and Kivikoski, A.: The significance of oestrogen activity in postmenopausal genital carcinoma. Annls Chir. Gynaec. Fenn. *53:* 110–114 (1964).

381 Rickford, R.B.K. and Whapham, E.M.: Benign ovarian neoplasms and postmenopausal haemorrhage. J. Obstet. Gynaec. Br. Emp. *49:* 653–659 (1942).

382 Roddick, J.W. and Greene, R.R.: The relation of nonmalignant postmenopausal endometrial changes to ovarian morphology. Am. J. Obstet. Gynec. *75:* 235–239 (1958).

383 Rome, M.; Brown, J.B.; Mason, T.; Smith, M.A.; Laverty, C., and Fortune, D.: Oestrogen excretion and ovarian pathology in postmenopausal women with atypical hyperplasia, adenocarcinoma and mixed adenosquamous carcinoma of the endometrium. Br. J. Obstet. Gynaec. *84:* 88–97 (1977).

384 Rome, R.M.; Laverty, C.R., and Brown, J.B.: Ovarian tumours in postmenopausal women. J. Obstet. Gynaec. Br. Commonw. *80:* 984–991 (1973).

385 Sall, S.; Weingold, A.B.; Sonnenblick, B., and Stone, M.L.: The effect of vaginal bleeding on survival in ovarian carcinoma. Surgery Gynec. Obstet. *117:* 601–603 (1963).

386 Scully, R.E.: An unusual ovarian tumor containing Leydig cells but associated with endometrial hyperplasia, in a postmenopausal woman. J. clin. Endocr. Metab. *13:* 1254–1263 (1953).

387 Sonwalker, A.: A study of urinary excretion. J. postgrad. Med. *20:* 103–106 (1974).

388 Stabnick, J.S.: Granulosa cell tumor in an 80-year-old patient case. Memphis med. J. *15:* 82–84 (1940).

389 Stevens, M.L. and Plotka, E.D.: Functional lutein cyst in a postmenopausal woman. Obstet. Gynec., N.Y. 50: 27s–29s (1977).
390 Szathmary, Z.v.: Mit Granulosazelltumor zusammenhängende, ungewöhnlich hochgradige Uterushypertrophie bei einer 63jährigen Kranken. Zentbl. Gynäk. 59: 2477–2482 (1935).
391 Targett, C.S.: Estrogen excretion in cases of theca-granulosa cell tumor. Am. J. Obstet. Gynec. 199: 859–861 (1974).
392 Treite, P.: Über zwei Fälle von Thecazelltumoren als Ursache postklimakterischer Blutungen. Zentbl. Gynäk. 64: 877–884 (1940).
393 Vácha, K. a Kopečný, J.: Karzinom v makroskopicky nezměněném vaječníku. Čslká Gynek. 36: 405–407 (1971).
394 Wachtel, E. and Plester, J.A.: The vaginal smear as an aid to diagnosis of genital tract malignancy in women. J. Obstet. Gynaec. Br. Emp. 59: 323–326 (1952).
395 Wimpfheimer, S.: Theca cell tumor of the ovary in a 72-year-old woman. J. Mt Sinai Hosp. 12: 768–772 (1965).
396 Winsauer, H.J. and Manning, J.C.: A masculinizing tumor of the ovary in a postmenopausal woman. J. clin. Endocr. Metab. 9: 774–781 (1949).
397 Winter, G.F.; Häntsch, R. und Rotter-Pool, P.: Das hormonal beeinflusste Endometrium in der Menopause (ungewöhnliche hormonale Aktivität bei Ovarialtumoren). Acta endocr., Copenh. 23: 295–312 (1956).
398 Woodruff, J.D.; Williams, T.J., and Goldberg, B.: Hormone activity of the common ovarian neoplasm. Am. J. Obstet. Gynec. 87: 679–698 (1963).
399 Wren, B.G. and Frampton, J.: Oestrogenic activity associated with nonfeminizing ovarian tumours after the menopause. Br. med. J. 5361: 842–844 (1963).

Miscellaneous Articles

400 Benthin, W.: Myome in der Menopause. Dt. med. Wschr. 65: 41–44 (1939).
401 Kofler, E.: Über die Häufigkeit vorheriger Hysterektomien und/oder unilateraler Ovarektomie bei Frauen mit malignen Ovarialtumoren. Geburtsh. Frauenheilk. 32: 873–881 (1972).
402 Kyank, H.: Prophylaktische Gesichtspunkte bei der Indikationsstellung gynäkologischer Operationen. Zentbl. Gynäk. 95: 833–840 (1973).
403 Lau, H. und Steidel, P.: Die Seitigkeit von Ovarialtumoren. Zur Frage der karzinomprophylaktischen unilateralen Ovarektomie. Geburtsh. Frauenheilk. 24: 156–159 (1964).
404 Siddall, R.S. and Levine, B.: Ovarian tumor prophylaxis by left oophorectomy. Am. J. Obstet. Gynec. 72: 1025–1028 (1956).
405 Wagenbichler, P.; Frauendorfer, H. und Havelec, L.: Der Einfluss der Hysterektomie und der einseitigen Ovarektomie auf das Auftreten von Ovarialtumoren. Geburtsh. Frauenheilk. 32: 882–890 (1972).

Subject Index